WALD-CAMPBELL

CW00435371

THE ANAESTHESIA OSCE

© 1997
Greenwich Medical Media
507 The Linen Hall
162-168 Regent Street
London
W1R 5TB

ISBN 1 900151 60X

First Published 1997

Apart from any fair dealing for the purposes of research or private study, or criticism or review, as permitted under the UK Copyright Designs and Patents Act, 1988, this publication may not be reproduced, stored, or transmitted, in any form or by any means, without the prior permission in writing of the publishers, or in the case of reprographic reproduction only in accordance with the terms of the licences issued by the Copyright Licensing Agency in the UK, or in accordance with the terms of the licences issued by the appropriate Reproduction Rights Organization outside the UK. Enquiries concerning reproduction outside the terms stated here should be sent to the publishers at the London address printed above.

The publisher makes no representation, express or implied, with regard to the accuracy of the information contained in this book and cannot accept any legal responsibility or liability for any errors or omissions that may be made.

A catalogue record for this book is available from the British Library

Distributed worldwide by
Oxford University Press

Designed and Produced by
Derek Virtue, DataNet

Printed in Great Britain by
Ashford Colour Press

THE ANAESTHESIA OSCE

K Eggers FRCA
J Everatt FRCA
SENIOR REGISTRARS
Welsh School of Anaesthesia
Maelor Hospital, Wrexham

G Arthurs FRCA
CONSULTANT ANAESTHETIST
Maelor Hospital, Wrexham

Illustrations by
T Bailey RGN RMN Cert Ed
Maelor Hospital, Wrexham

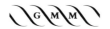

CONTENTS

4 PHYSICAL EXAMINATION

5 COMMUNICATION

6 RESUSCITATION

7 APPARATUS

ANSWERS

8 ECG

ANSWERS

9 X-RAYS

ANSWERS

INTRODUCTION

The objective structured clinical examination (OSCE) is a good way of examining a candidate's abilities over a range of skills and reduces examiner bias. The OSCE can assess skills that have not previously been tested, such as the ability to communicate with, or give advice to patients.

The purpose of this book is to help candidates practise for the OSCE and at the same time encourage the development of skills such as communication and history taking that are essential to a good clinician. An anaesthetist is a doctor first and then an anaesthetist. A knowledge of both the way to effectively communicate with patients and good history taking is as important as being able to site an epidural catheter or a tracheal tube.

When you enter the examination premises there is a cloak room for hanging coats but you will need to carry your identification card, wallet and a stethoscope with you, so wear clothes with pockets or carry a bag. Think about wearing clothes that will allow you to kneel on the floor in the resuscitation station.

The OSCE is made up of a number of quite separate stations. The guidance in: "The Royal College of Anaesthetists Examinations Regulations" should be read for more details. The regulations indicate that there will be 16 stations lasting approximately 2 hours. Each station is of 5 minutes duration with a 90 second break between stations. There are at least two rest stations which are also of 5 minutes each with a 90 second preliminary break making a total of six and a half minutes rest. Drinking water is provided at the rest station as candidates may become quite dry and thirsty with talking for this period of time. In the 90 second break you will sit in a small booth. There will be a notice with the title of the next station and a short introduction. Read these notes carefully and consider how you will approach this station. Each station is marked to give a score for that station. This mark is quite separate from all the other stations. It is necessary to gain a pass mark in most of the stations in order to pass the whole examination. The marks from one station are not added to those in another station. All stations carry equal marks. Some stations may be marked with a point subtracted for a wrong answer, as in the MCQ examination. Check carefully at each examination for which, if any, of the stations have negative marking. If there is no negative marking guess, if there is negative marking be more careful.

At the beginning of the examination each candidate is briefed and then directed to a particular booth which is the waiting place before their first station. When every one is in their correct place a bell or whistle sounds and you move to the station. However hyper-adrenergic you feel read carefully the instructions for the first station you are about to enter. Some candidates will be in the booth before the rest station and will start the examination with a rest. Equally some will finish at a rest station. Be prepare to start anywhere in the circuit. Use each rest booth to clear your mind of the previous station and do not let one poor performance spoil the next station. The role of the examiner varies between stations. At some an examiner will be observing your performance, at others the examiner will ask you questions and at others you will be left to fill in an answer sheet with minimum examiner contact.

We would emphasis that we feel that one way to failure is not to practise. Stations which involve talking to, or examining a patient particularly require practise if only to perform the task in five minutes. Have a system or order and apply it methodically so as not to miss out anything. Do not fail to ask simple questions like: "Why are you in hospital?", "What are you worried about and why?". "Do you smoke or drink"?". For history taking and communication ask a friend to act the part. You may not like the idea of role play but you will meet it in the examination so find a fellow candidate and use each other. We have drawn computer generated figures, chest x-rays and apparatus diagrams for better black and white reproduction. The actual OSCE will have actual apparatus, proper chest x-rays and ECGs but with identification removed.

The type of stations that may be examined are:

Resuscitation

To demonstrate how to resuscitate a collapsed adult or child. The recommendations of the Resuscitation Council should be followed exactly.

Communication skills

The skills required here are to listen carefully to the patient and identify the problem(s). Then a number of approaches may be relevant: to give a comprehensive explanation of the problem, to explain a procedure, to reassure a patient about their anxieties, to obtain consent or to talk about a medical problem. While some time must be spent listening to ensure that you are on the correct topic it is also important to give accurate and adequate explanations. There may be two of these stations.

History taking

Take a comprehensive and relevant history from the patient.

Relevant in this context means: identifying the main and secondary condition(s) from which the patient is suffering; the reason for surgery and the fitness of the patient for that surgery; possible anaesthetic or peri-operative problems.

There may be two of these stations.

The follow on station

This follows after the history taking station. It concerns the examinations and investigations that might be relevant to aid the diagnosis of the patient that you have just interviewed at the history taking station. Also included are general questions about the condition, drug therapy or management of the patient peri-operatively.

Apparatus

The apparatus may need testing or setting up. There may be pictures with questions based on an MCQ pattern. Practise checking all anaesthetic equipment including the anaesthetic machine. We have presented the reader with a number of apparatus quizzes.

Skill station

This usually involves a piece of apparatus and the ability to perform a skill such as crico-thyroid puncture or the use of an epidural catheter.

Data interpretation

There will probably be a set of results and 10 questions on those results at each station. There will be a number of these stations, each one on a different aspect of clinical information, i.e. there will not be two of the same item. There might be tests of knowledge about CXR, ECG, plasma haematology, electrolytes, arterial gases, pulmonary and cardiac function and anything else that can be investigated relevant to the clinical situation. Check for negative marking. If there is no negative marking then try all the questions.

Clinical examination

This involves demonstrating how you will examine part of a patient. This might be one system, e.g. the respiratory system; part of a system, e.g. certain cranial or peripheral nerves; or one particular physiological measurement, e.g. the blood pressure with some questions relevant to blood pressure.

DATA INTERPRETATION 1

INTRODUCTION

Each station involving data interpretation is laid out with an artefact or set of results. The artefact may be an ECG or CXR and the set of results from such tests as: haematology, biochemistry, lung function and cardiac catheter studies. First study the essential information that is given. There will be an answer sheet on which you mark your answers, similar to an MCQ sheet but with more questions. All questions will be answerable as Yes/No or True/False.

DATA 1

(Answers on page 11)

A patient presents with the following haematological results (normal values in brackets):

Haemoglobin 10 g/dl	(11.5-16.5)
PCV 0.3	(0.4-0.55)
RBC 3 x 10^{12}/l	(4.5-6.0)
Reticulocytes 0.3% of RBC	(0-2%)
Platelets 90 x 10^9/l	(150-400)
WBC 5.6 x 10^9/l	(4-11)

Questions

1. – The red cells might show anisocytosis.   True   False

2. – The patient has a MCV of 100 fl   True   False

3. – The patient has a MCH of 28 pg.   True   False

4. – This anaemia is seen in pregnant patients.   True   False

5. – The serum B_{12} and folate should be measured.   True   False

6. – The patient might complain of a sore tongue.   True   False

7. – The administration of nitrous oxide for 6 hours
       causes changes to cells in the bone marrow.   True   False

8. – Ferrous sulphate could be given to treat this patient.   True   False

9. – If the patient is blood group AB they could safely
       receive a transfusion of SAGM blood group A.   True   False

10. – Blood transfusion reduces the incidence of
        rejection of some organs.   True   False

DATA 2
(Answers on page 12)

A 67 year old patient has had several episodes of paroxysmal nocturnal dyspnoea. The cardiac catheter studies show the following pressures (mmHg):

	Phasic	Mean
Right atrium	–	12
Right ventricle	60/5	–
Pulmonary artery	60/30	40
Pulmonary artery wedge	–	27
Left atrium	40/20	
Left ventricle	120/0	–
LVEDP	0	
Aorta	120/60	

Questions

1. – The right atrial pressure is normal.   True   False

2. – The pulmonary valve is stenosed.   True   False

3. – Pulmonary oedema is likely to be present.   True   False

4. – There will be a diastolic murmur.   True   False

5. – There is likely to be a systolic murmur.   True   False

6. – The mitral valve normally has an area of 7 cm².   True   False

7. – The patient has aortic valve disease.   True   False

8. – This condition is most commonly seen in females with a history of rheumatic fever.   True   False

9. – Echocardiography can be used to assess left ventricular hypertrophy.   True   False

10. – In this patient the difference in pressure between the left ventricle and left atrium is proportional to the degree of disease.   True   False

DATA 3

(Answers on page 13)

A 75 years old lady receiving an oral hypoglycaemic and diet to control her diabetes is admitted following 24 hours of nausea and vomiting with abdominal pain suggestive of appendicitis. Normal values are given in brackets.

Sodium	140 mmol/l	(136-149)
Potassium	5 mmol/l	(3.8-5.2)
Bicarbonate	8 mmol/l	(24-30)
Chloride	98 mmol/l	(100-107)
P_aO_2	13 kPa on air	(12-15)
P_aCO_2	2.4 kPa	(4.5-6.1)
pH	7.1	(7.4)
Glucose	30 mmol/l	(3.0-5.3)
Urea	15 mmol/l	(2.5-6.6)

Questions

1. – The patient has a respiratory acidosis.	True	False
2. – There is an anion gap of 39 mmol/l.	True	False
3. – The normal anion gap is less than 18 mmol/l.	True	False
4. – The patient's condition is compatible with a non-ketotic hyper-osmolar state.	True	False
5. – The ECG will show small P waves.	True	False
6. – A urine osmolarity of 200 mosmol/l is only found with prerenal failure.	True	False
7. – Initial treatment should include calcium.	True	False
8. – Glucose and insulin would be a safe combination to administer to this patient.	True	False
9. – Dehydration alone could account for this urea concentration.	True	False
10. – The calculated serum osmolarity is 355 mosmol/l.	True	False

DATA 4

(Answers on page 14)

A 62 year old man complains of breathlessness. Lung function tests show:

> FVC 2.4 l (predicted 2.4 to 3.6)
> FEV$_1$ 1.4 l
> RV 2.8 l (predicted 1.6 to 2.3)
> FRC 3.4 l (predicted 2.2 to 3.3)
> TLC 5.9 l (predicted 3.9 to 5.6)
> TLCO 4.5 mmol/min/kPa (predicted 5.8 to 8.7)
> KCO 0.8 mmol/min/kPa/l

The vitalograph and siprometer trace are shown opposite.

Questions

1. – FEV$_1$ is the volume of gas breathed out in a normal breath.   True   False

2. – The results are compatible with obstructive lung disease.   True   False

3. – The TLC can be measured using a vitalograph.   True   False

4. – The tests are compatible with emphysema.   True   False

5. – Steroids might benefit this patient.   True   False

6. – Propranolol may improve this lung function.   True   False

7. – This picture can be caused by ankylosing spondylitis.   True   False

8. – The ECG may show tall P waves.   True   False

9. – The vitalograph trace represents the figures in the data.   True   False

10. – The spirometer trace is correctly labelled.   True   False

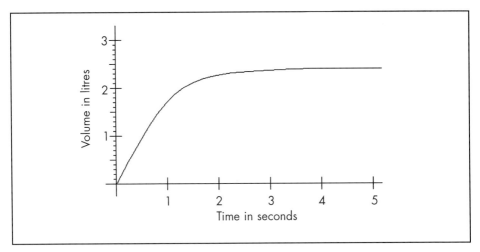

Vitalograph

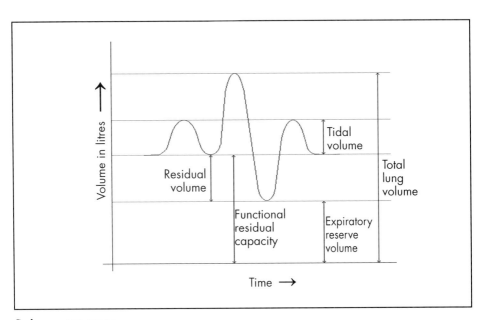

Spirometer trace

DATA 5

(Answers on page 15)

A patient is breathless before routine surgery. Pulse and blood pressure are normal. Arterial blood gases show (normal values are given in brackets):

pH 7.55	
P_aO_2 8 kPa breathing air.	
Aterial blood saturation 90%	
P_aCO_2 3.5 kPa	
Bicarbonate 20 mmol/l	(24–30)
BEB –4	(0)
Hb 15 g/dl	(11.5–16.5)

Questions

1. – The patient will be centrally cyanosed at rest. True False

2. – The patient will benefit from oxygen by face mask. True False

3. – The results are suggestive of a metabolic
   keto-acidosis. True False

4. – This is an acute situation. True False

5. – A possible diagnosis would be pulmonary emboli. True False

6. – The patient will benefit from doxapram therapy. True False

7. – If the patient is a cigarette smoker the pulse
   oximeter will under-read the oxygen saturation. True False

8. – Correcting the alkalosis will lower the oxygen
   saturation at the same P_aO_2. True False

9. – The arterial oxygen content is about 18 ml/100 ml. True False

10. – The patient should be limited to low concentrations
    of inspired oxygen. True False

DATA 6

(Answers on page 16)

The following results are from a preoperative patient (normal values are given in brackets).

Bilirubin 186 μmol/l	(3–18)
Aspartate transaminase 120 i.u./l	(5–30)
Albumin 35 g/l	(35–50)
Calcium (total) 2.14 mmol/l	(2.25–2.6)
Alkaline phosphatase 600 i.u./l	(17–100)
Gamma-glutamyl transpeptidase 25 i.u./l	(10–55)
Urine Positive for conjugated bilirubin.	

Questions

1. – The patient would appear clinically jaundiced.   True   False

2. – These findings are typical of alcoholic liver disease.   True   False

3. – These findings could be due to gall stones.   True   False

4. – These findings are typical of a patient with hepatitis A.   True   False

5. – The absence of pain suggests the presence of a carcinoma.   True   False

6. – In a preoperative coagulation screen the partial thromboplastin time (PTT) would be a sensitive measurement of the degree of liver impairment.   True   False

7. – The serum albumin will indicate whether there is chronically impaired liver function.   True   False

8. – Correction of any coagulopathy in this patient should be with cryoprecipitate.   True   False

9. – 10 mg of vitamin K should be administered daily until 3 days after the operation.   True   False

10. – The prevention of peri-operative renal failure in such a patient should include the administration of mannitol or frusemide.   True   False

DATA 7

(Answers on page 17)

Pulmonary catheter pressures.

Questions

1. – Label the site of the pulmonary artery flotation catheter at each position A to D on the diagram opposite.

2. – The right ventricular pressure is abnormal. True False

3. – Pulmonary oedema can be present with a normal pulmonary wedge pressure. True False

4. – The average value for oxygen delivery to the tissues in a healthy adult at rest is 1500 ml/min. True False

5. – The average oxygen consumption for an adult at rest is 250 ml/min. True False

6. – Increasing the F_iO_2 from 20% to 100% in a healthy person will increase the delivery of oxygen by 25%. True False

7. – Systemic vascular resistance can be calculated by using the equation:

(mean arterial pressure – central venous pressure) x 80 divided by cardiac output.

or

(MAP - CVP) x 80 / CO. True False

8. – The systemic vascular resistance is reduced by sepsis. True False

9. – Pulmonary vascular resistance is reduced by hypoxia. True False

10. – Pulmonary vascular resistance is high in cor pulmonale. True False

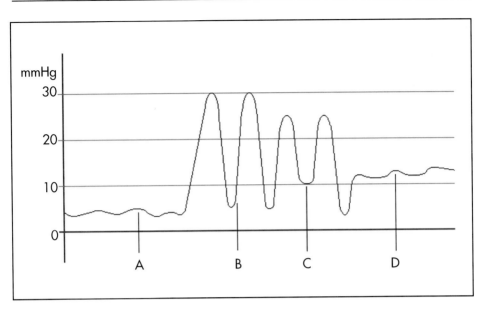

ANSWERS
DATA INTERPRETATION

Answers – Data 1

1. True – Anisocytosis is a variation in red cell size often seen with anaemia.

2. True – The MCV (mean corpuscular volume) is PCV/RBC (in this case 0.3/3). Under 76 fl (fl = femto or 10^{-15}) – microcytic cells, over 95 fl – macrocytic cells.

3. False – MCH is Hb/RBC, here 10/3= 33 pg (normal 27 to 32 pg, p=picogram pico = 10^{-12}).

4. True – Macrocytosis may be due to
- deficiency of folate e.g. diet, pregnancy, cell breakdown as in leukaemia, drugs like anti-convulsants;
- B_{12} deficiency e.g. pernicious anaemia and lack of intrinsic factor, following gastrectomy, blind loop syndrome, ileal disease, tape worm;
- Other reasons e.g. liver disease and alcoholism, myxoedema and following heamorrhage associated with a raised reticulocyte count.

5. True – The patient has a macrocytic anaemia – MCV 100 fl.

6. True – Patients with pernicious anaemia have sore tongues, dyspepsia, neurological disorders, liver enlargement and retinal haemorrhages and may have gastric carcinoma. There is an association with certain autoimmune conditions like myasthenia gravis and thyrotoxicosis.

7. True – Nitrous oxide exposure causes inhibition of methionine synthetase activity which will lead in time to megaloblastic changes.

8. False – This is not an iron deficiency anaemia.

9. True – AB is a rare group (3% population), with A and B antigen on the red cells but no serum antibodies. Group A is common (45% population) with A antigen on the red cells and antibodies to B in the serum. These antibodies are washed away in the formation of SAGM blood.

10. True – The incidence of kidney rejection is reduced. The recurrence of some cancer cells may be increased.

Answers – Data 2

1. **False** – Normal 0-7mmHg.

2. **False** – No pressure gradient from the right ventricle to the pulmonary artery.

3. **True** – A wedge pressure above 15mmHg may be associated with pulmonary oedema.

4. **True** – There is mitral stenosis. The PAWP is about the same as the left atrial pressure and at the end of diastole PAWP is higher than LV diastolic pressure.

5. **True** – There are two reasons why this patient is likely to have a systolic murmur:-

   • Mitral stenosis due to rheumatic heart disease is likely to be associated with mitral incompetance with the high left atrial pressure.

   • The high pulmonary arterial pressure suggests the development of pulmonary hypertension which will lead to right ventricular failure, dilatation and tricuspid incompetance.

6. **False** – Normally 5cm^2.

7. **False** – The pressures and gradient across the aortic valve are normal.

8. **True** – Mitral stenosis is commonest in women following rheumatic fever.

9. **True** – Echocardiography would indicate the size or diameter of the left ventricle. At the end of diastole a diameter of over 55 mm would mean that myocardial function is likely to remain impaired even after valve replacement. Another indicator of impaired left ventricular function is end diastolic pressure. A pressure greater than 20 mmHg suggests severe impairment to left ventricular function.

10. **True** – The gradient is proportional to the degree of the stenosis.

Answers – Data 3

1. **False** – Metabolic acidosis: low pH, low CO_2. with a compensatory respiratory alkalosis.

2. **True** – The anion gap in the total of all the positive ions (cations) minus the total of all the negative ions (anions).

3. **True** – Anion gap: Difference between anions and cations should be no more than 17 mmol/l. An anion gap approaching 40 implies a severe metabolic acidosis, e.g. severe ketoacidosis.

4. **False** – Non-ketotic hyper-osmolar states have a lower anion gap but a higher osmolarity of over 360 mosmol/l. The biguanide oral hypoglycaemic, metformin, can induce a lactic acidosis in patients if taken in overdose, or in the presence of hepatic or renal failure.

5. **?.False** – The ECG with hypokalaemia shows ST depression, T wave flattening or inversion, prominent U waves which may combine with the P wave to enlarge it. Hyperkalaemia gives small P wave and tall peaked T waves. The QRS will widen and the patient is at risk from ventricular fibrillation.

6. **False** – A urine osmolarity of 200 mosmol/l implies the inability to concentrate within the kidney. It also occurs with the passing of very dilute urine as in diabetes insipidus.

7. **False** – There is no point in giving calcium.

8. **False** – The serum potassium will fall if potassium is not given with the glucose and insulin.

9. **True** – Urea is raised in dehydration due to reduced elimination. This raised urea is not specific to dehydration. Other causes are renal dysfunction and increased protein absoption e.g. with a gastrointestinal bleed.

   To assess the degree of dehydration the serum albumin can be used if liver function is normal.

   To assesss renal function serum creatinine can be used assuming that muscle breakdown is normal as creatinine depends only on renal elimination.

10. **False** – The calculated osmolarity is given by: $Na + K + Cl + HCO_3 + urea + glucose = 140 + 5 + 98 + 8 + 30 + 15 = $ total 296 mosmol/l. A deduction of osmolarity can be made by $2 \times (Na + K) + (urea) + (glucose)$. This assumes that the number of anions equals the number of cations.

Answers – Data 4

1. **False** – The volume breathed out in the first second of a forced expiration.

2. **True** – The tests show a reduced FEV_1 to FVC ratio (normal >70%) and a hyperinflated lung.

3. **False** – TLC is measured using helium dilution or whole body plethysmography.

4. **True** – The hyperinflated lung and the reduced carbon monoxide transfer factor are typical of emphysema.

5. **True** – The patient might also benefit from oxygen, and a bronchodilator such as a $beta_2$ adrenoreceptor agonist (salbutalmol or terbutaline) or an anti-muscarinic (ipatropium).

6. **False** – Beta blockers are contraindicated as they may aggravate bronchospasm

7. **False** – Ankylosing spondylitis is associated with restrictive lung disease. This pattern of obstructive airways disease can be caused by chronic smoking, living in an environment polluted with dust, cadmium poisoning, $alpha_1$ antitrypsin deficiency (homozygous), MacLeod's syndrome, Bullous disease of lung, Kartagener's syndrome.

8. **True** – As a sign of right artrial enlargement. P pulmonale results from right atrial enlargement which occurs secondary to pulmonary hypertension from hypoxic pulmonary vasoconstriction

9. **True** –

10. **False** – The residual volume and expiratory reserve volume have been swapped around.

Answers – Data 5

1. **False** – Central cyanosis will normally occur when the P_aO_2 is <6kPa. Central cyanosis requires 5 g/dl of reduced haemoglobin. Peripheral cyanosis depends on local perfusion.

2. **True** – The patient has a reduced arterial carbon dioxide tension and so does not depend on hypoxia to drive respiration. Oxygen therapy will raise the arterial oxygen tension and saturation.

3. **False** – A respiratory alkalosis is present.

4. **False** – The results are suggestive of a chronic, compensated respiratory alkalosis with a low carbon dioxide and a compensatory reduced bicarbonate ion.

5. **True** – The patient has a reduced oxygen saturation breathing air. This could be due to a ventilation to perfusion mismatch. Possible causes are: Pulmonary emboli, lung infection and consolidation, pulmonary oedema. A right to left cardiac shunt could also cause this hypoxia.

6. **False** – The respiratory drive is intact.

7. **False** – Carboxyhaemoglobin will be present, half of which will be read as oxyhaemoglobin, giving an over-reading of true oxyhaemoglobin.

8. **True** – The oxygen dissociation curve is shifted to the right by increasing acidosis or reducing alkalosis.

9. **True** – Oxygen content = Hb g/dl x saturation x 1.34 ml/g = 18.09 ml/ 100 ml.

10. **False** – Patients with type I respiratory failure (pink puffers), such as this patient, have a low or normal P_aCO_2 and do not depend on their hypoxic drive for respiration.

    Those patients with type II respiratory failure (blue bloaters) have a high P_aCO_2 and depend on a hypoxic drive to maintain respiration.

Answers – Data 6

1. **True** – The bilirubin is over 40 μmol/l.

2. **False** – Gamma-glutamyl transpeptidase is low. The MCV may also be increased in alcoholic liver disease.

3. **True** – Alkaline phosphatase is raised. This indicates biliary obstruction. The causes of obstruction are gall stones, drugs e.g. contraceptives, carcinoma of the pancreas and primary biliary cirrhosis.

4. **False** – AST too low. The AST would be very high in any acute hepatitis.

5. **True** – No pain suggests carcinoma of the pancreas. Pain suggests cholecystitis, biliary duct obstruction due to gall stones or a distended liver capsule.

6. **False** – Prothrombin time (PT) is better as it relies on the liver produced clotting factors 2,7,9,10.

7. **True** – As the liver is the sole source of albumin production a low albumin would suggest chronic liver impairment.

8. **False** – Vitamin K or fresh frozen plasma should be considered.

9. **True**

10. **True** – The risk of peri-operative renal failure will be reduced by good hydration, mannitol, frusemide and dopamine.

Answers – Data 7

1. – A. Right atrium, B. Right ventricle, C. Pulmonary artery, D. Catheter in wedge position.

2. **False** – The right ventriclar pressure is normally within the range of 15-25/ 0-8 mmHg.

3. **True** – If the alveolar endothelim is damaged or if the serum osmotic pressure is low.

4. **False** – Cardiac output is 5000 ml/min and oxygen content 20 ml/100 ml. The average value for oxygen delivery to the tissues in a healthy adult at rest is 1000 ml/min. The true delivery of oxygen to the tissues at rest is given by the equation:

    Oxygen delivery = cardiac output x ((arterial oxygen saturation x haemoglobin concentration x 1.34) + (partial pressure of arterial oxygen x 0.023)) divided by 100.

    or

    DO_2 ml/min = CO ml/min x ((S_aO_2/100 x Hb g/dl x 1.39) + (P_aO_2 kPa x 0.023)) / 100.

5. **True**

6. **False** – Most of the oxygen is carried by the haemoglobin. The only increase will be in dissolved oxygen at the rate of 0.023ml/100ml blood/kPa.

7. **True** – Calculated as 1000-2000 dynes sec/cm^5. 80 is a correction factor.

8. **True** – SVR is reduced by vasodilators, volatile anaesthetic agents, regional anaesthesia, and anaphylatic, septic and neurogenic shock.

9. **False** – Pulmonary vascular resistance is reduced by nitric oxide and prostacyclin. It is increased by hypoxia and acidosis.

10. **True** – Hypoxic pulmonary vasoconstriction occurs secondary to chronic lung disease leading to cor pulmonale. It is also high in VSD with Eisenmenger's syndrome which can occur in Down's syndrome patients. Its importance is the possibility of a worsening in the reverse shunt with IPPV.

HISTORY TAKING **2**

INTRODUCTION

There is a finite amount of time in which to obtain all the facts that you require. In the OSCE this is 5 minutes. Limit yourself to taking a history; do not start to examine the pulse, or explain a symptom as part of history taking. You should be prepared to identify yourself by your number to the examiners. With the patient start by introducing yourself by name. In the past no candidate's name was spoken in the examination but candidates now have to carry an identification badge and you should speak to the patient as you would in a real clinical situation. Then ask about the presenting complaint: *"What operation are you to have, which side is it?"* *"What is your main complaint, how long have you had the problem, when did it start or what started the complaint?"* Anaesthetists are doctors first so explore the present complaint before asking about problems with previous anaesthetics. The present complaint may give you the lead into further questions e.g. vascular problems, cataracts and diabetes, arthritis and neck movement. Allow the patient a few seconds to tell his or her story. Do not cut across the story too early, you may miss a vital piece of information. As the history unfolds think of further questions or side issues. Try to ask open ended questions. These are questions that cannot be answered by Yes or No. For instance: *"Tell me about your symptoms?"* *"Where do you get pain?"*. *"What other operations have you had?"* **Not:** *"Did you have an operation in the past?"* Answer: "Yes." or "No."

Construct an order to your questioning after you have obtained the details of the main problem.

One order is:

* Present complaint,
* Past medical history,
* Past anaesthetic/operative history
  – ask about problems with teeth, regurgitation,
  veins, DVT, airway, pain relief and PONV,
* Drug and allergy history,
* Social history: age, job and country of origin or travel history,
  smoking habits, alcohol intake and social drugs.
* Family illnesses.

After exploring the main problem in all its facets conduct a survey of each relevant system of the body, such as: cardiovascular, respiratory, renal, hepatic, neurological and allergies. In depth, anaesthetic related questions, such as difficulty with airway, will normally be part of another OSCE. Remember that in an examination it is possible for a patient to have a second, possibly unrelated problem, or a twist to the history. In real life you hope that the patient only has one problem; do not assume this about the person in the OSCE.

Think of relationships: If there have been previous operations: what were they, were there any problems? Gastrectomy may be followed by anaemia due to diet or mega-loblastic changes related to loss of intrinsic factor. Thyroidectomy patients may have an increased or reduced thyroid function as well as a recurrent laryngeal nerve lesion from surgery. Hernia patients may have an associated intra-abdominal tumour. Patients with diabetes and rheumatoid arthritis may have problems with many systems.

Explore medications for a history of their side effects as well as any recent changes in prescribing.

Smokers may have lung cancer and smoking is associated with drinking alcohol which may lead to oesophageal varices or liver disease. There is a relationship between drugs of addiction and alcohol. Do not forget to ask about alcohol intake. Certain jobs are associated with diseases; such as asbestosis in the building trade, cancer of the bladder in the dye industry, dust diseases of the lung from mining and farmer's lung. It may be relevant to ask about drug habits, exposure to hepatitis and possible AIDS infection. Anyone can be affected, so if in doubt ask: "*Do you use drugs other than for your health, do you use drugs for social reasons?*" or, "*Are you at risk from having AIDS or Hepatitis (have you had yellow jaundice)?*"

In each of the histories that follow there is an opening statement. Then the history develops with a number of questions. Try to answer each question before moving to the next stage. Compare your decisions with the commentary to see if you have picked up the issues that may be important. You may ask a friend to act each part by reading the scenario summary at the beginning of the answer for each section together with the questions and answers. Give yourself exactly five minutes and see what you have missed out.

Each history station is followed by a "follow on station". The "follow on" is related to what has been said at the preceding history taking. It may involve asking for relevant tests and explaining the results. You should be in the habit of only asking for a test if you have a reason for the request. If the patient has been bleeding it is logical to request a full blood count, but it is difficult to request a chest x-ray if there are no respiratory symptoms, no evidence of tumour, tuberculosis or smoking. There may then follow questions about the specific condition that the patient suffers from, medication or related medical or anaesthetic problems.

HISTORY 1

(Answers on page 31)

You are asked to see a man of 67 years for a cystoscopy as a day patient.

Questions

1. – Write down what you consider are the important issues in the history that you will ask the patient about – specific to the introduction you have been given.

Introduce yourself by name, followed by a history of the cystoscopy.

2. – What will you ask?

The patient says he has haematuria.

3. – What are the causes of haematuria and what are the follow up questions that should be asked?

4. – How can you differentiate between acute and chronic blood loss?

Any patient coming for a cystoscopy should have their renal function assessed.

5. – What will you ask to assess renal function?

6. – What are the relevant points about being a day case?

7. – What else should you have asked about?

FOLLOW ON STATION 1 (*Answers on page 33*)

If you have not taken a full history you will have problems at the follow on station which will be concerned with topics such as relevant investigations and treatment.

An examiner might ask the following questions. You probably do not lose points for guessing, only time.

Questions

1. – This patient is found to have a haemoglobin of 9 g/dl. This is likely to be due to an obstructive uropathy.   True   False

2. – The anaemia could be linked to a previous gastrectomy.   True   False

3. – This patient should be transfused pre-operatively for a routine cystoscopy.   True   False

4. – The patient is found to be a hepatitis B carrier. He could have been infected from his mother.   True   False

5. – Hepatitis A leads to liver cirrhosis.   True   False

6. – Over half of the population over 50 years have IgG antibodies to HAV.   True   False

7. – A creatinine of 150 μmol/l is probably due to a muscle wasting disease.   True   False

8. – The loss of 500 ml of blood will lead to a 10% reduction in blood pressure in a healthy male.   True   False

9. – A normochromic, normocytic anaemia suggests chronic renal disease.   True   False

10. – A measure of the volume of a 24 hour urine output will be a useful guide to this patient's renal function.   True   False

HISTORY 2

(Answers on page 34)

You are asked to see a lady of 79 years old who is on your list for an elective hysterectomy.

Introduce yourself by name.

Questions

1. − What issues might be relevant to start with?

The hysterectomy is for post menopausal bleeding.

2. − What follow up questions does this suggest?

3. − How will you assess the amount of blood loss leading to possible anaemia?

This patient suffers from syncope and has recently been prescribed an ACE inhibitor for hypertension.

4. − What do you want to know?

Does the patient take other drugs?

5. − She takes aspirin - why and for what effect?

The patient now says she is also taking warfarin.

6. − Why is she taking warfarin and what difference does this make to your history?

7. − Finally what else will you check for?

FOLLOW ON STATION 2

(Answers on page 36)

Questions

1-5. – Give five test results you would like to see and *why*?

6. – What changes will you make before surgery?

7. – Name at least four explanations for the falling.

8. – If the patient had a haemoglobin of 9 g/100 ml would you routinely transfuse her pre-operatively?

9. – Can you explain how the amount of oxygen delivered to the tissues varies with different haemoglobin concentrations?

HISTORY 3

(Answers on page 38)

You are told that at the next station you should take a history from the patient who is to have a thyroidectomy.

Questions

1. – How will you start your history taking?

2. – What symptoms of thyroid disease will you explore in the history?

You decide that the symptoms suggest hyperthyroidism.

3. – What drug history would you ask about?

4. – What associated conditions will you ask about?

The patient indicates that they had an episode of chest pain and hospital admission 4 weeks ago.

5. – What are the possible causes of chest pain and what treatment might follow?

6. – What general questions will you ask?

FOLLOW ON STATION 3 *(Answers on page 39)*

Questions

1-4. – What four investigations would you like to be done and what results might they give?

5. – How can you distinguish clinically between hyperthyroidism and anxiety?

6. – What structure(s) must be protected during surgery?

7. – What is the beneficial effect to this patient of taking aspirin?

8. – Name four side effects of aspirin therapy.

9. – Name two immediate postoperative complications peculiar to thyroidectomy.

10. – Name two later complications peculiar to thyroidectomy.

HISTORY 4 *(Answers on page 40)*

You are to take a history from a lady who is to have an arthroscopy.

Questions

1. – How will you start?

The main symptom is a "wheeze or bad chest".
The patient might indicate that they have an inhaler.

2. – How will you explore this symptom?

This lady has had a chest problem since childhood.

3. – What could be the cause of this scenario?
   What treatment could have been given that might be related in the history?

There are many causes of breathlessness.

4. – How will you differentiate the types of breathlessness from the history?

5. – In what ways may the patient's job have a bearing on the present symptoms?

6. – What extra points might be relevant?

FOLLOW ON STATION 4 (Answers on page 42)

Questions

1-3. – What three investigations would you like to see the results from, giving one reason for performing each test?

You have to justify asking for each test.

4. – Pre-operatively this patient should have prophylactic benzylpenicillin.   True   False

5. – What does a FEV_1 of 1.5 litres and a FVC of 3.5 litres suggest?

6. – What treatment is indicated?

7. – If the patient has had a recent haemoptysis what further investigation should be performed?

8, 9. – What two treatments would you prescribe postoperatively for this patient?

10. – If the patient is on steroids what dose regime would you use post-operatively?

HISTORY 5

(Answers on page 43)

You are asked to take a relevant history from a patient who has arthritis. She is to have a cholecystectomy.

Start by introducing yourself and asking about her main symptoms.

Questions

1. – What are the lines of enquiry you will follow?

2. – What types of arthritis may she have and how will you question her to determine which she has?

You decide that this lady has rheumatoid arthritis.

3. – What do you need to know about?

4. – Which drugs will you enquire about and why?

The operation is to be a cholecystectomy.

5. – What symptoms will she have had and what is the differential diagnosis?

The patient indicates that she has diabetes mellitus.

6. – What do you need to explore about diabetes?

FOLLOW ON STATION 5 *(Answers on page 45)*

A laparoscopic cholecystectomy is planned.

Questions

1 - 4. – Which four investigations would you like the results from?

    5. – If the patient is jaundiced during the 3 days before operation name 2 precautions that should be taken.

    6. – Rheumatoid arthritis is a disease of the synovium.   True   False

    7. – The commonest anaemia in rheumatoid arthritis is a hypochromic anaemia.   True   False

    8. – An insulin dependent diabetic should receive an infusion of glucose pre-operatively and an infusion of glucose and insulin postoperatively.   True   False

    9. – The blood glucose should be monitored every thirty minutes during the operation.   True   False

  10. – During laparoscopy a pneumothorax, containing carbon dioxide, can develop without trauma to the thorax wall.   True   False

ANSWERS
HISTORY TAKING

Answers – HISTORY 1

Scenario: Man, with haematuria, has had several cystoscopies for haematuria but recently has had a bigger bleed than usual and comes as a day patient for another cystoscopy.

1. You will want to explore the reasons for the cystoscopy. What symptoms, when did they first occur, how long has he had symptoms for? Also, is he suitable for day care?

2. Check through possible reasons for having a cystoscopy?
   a. for poor urine flow - prostatism.
   b. haematuria.
   c. incontinence.
   d. dysuria or pain due to infection.
   e. incontinence - urethral valves.

3. Haematuria
   a. clotting disorder:
      i. congenital – haemophilia.
      ii. acquired – anticoagulants, bone marrow disorders, liver disease: does the patient bruise easily or bleed excessively when cut? (Adult causes of a clotting defect ? Think of conditions invading the bone marrow. Liver disease linked to a high alcohol intake.)
   b. infection in bladder or kidney: pain in loin or dysuria.
   c. tumour: bladder, benign papilloma or cancer; renal tract or kidney. Ask about job - dye workers get bladder cancer and pain.
   d. prostate disease: tumour or infection: altered stream, nocturia and frequency, pain dysuria or secondaries give bone pain.
   e. stones: family history, travel to hot climates. Pain in loin, along line of ureter, on passing urine.

   Loss of weight, general ill health or febrile episodes suggest: cancer or infection, may be primary, or secondary to tumour or obstruction to urine flow.

   Check that this is haematuria: from urethra/penis - in the urine? Could it be from the rectum or vagina in a woman?

4. Symptoms of blood loss.

   a. How much blood have you lost? Over what period of time? The amount may be reflected in whether the patient felt tiredness or syncope.

   b. When did you lose blood? Is it a sudden, acute loss or chronic, or acute on chronic?

The effect of acute blood loss depends on the amount of blood loss and the time since the loss. Immediately afterwards there are no changes in the haematocrit but changes in the CVS. A loss of 10% will lead to a tachycardia and vasoconstriction. A loss of 20% blood volume in a fit adult will often not be associated with hypotension. Hypotension becomes apparent with blood loss of 30% of blood volume or more. After a short period of time haemodilution occurs to recreate the circulating volume. Acute blood loss may be associated with syncope or the sudden onset of angina or breathlessness.

Chronic blood loss will allow time for physiological adjustment giving a normal circulating volume, normal heart rate and blood pressure but limited exercise tolerance. Chronic blood loss may lead to anaemia and oedema may develop.

Consider that you may be asked to explain the different red cell profiles and haematocrits that will occur in acute and chronic blood loss. Acute blood loss will initially show a normal haemoglobin concentration. PCV will depend on the resuscitation fluids. Chronic loss will lead to a low haemoglobin concentration, possibly iron deficiency anaemia and a raised reticulocyte count indicating increased turnover of erythrocytes. In contrast rheumatoid arthritis and chronic renal failure will show a normocytic normochromic anaemia.

5. Concentrating capacity may be reduced. This will present as polyuria and nocturia. Oedema from salt and water retention occurs in chronic renal failure, with hypertension. Poor stream and frequency are not necessarily renal symptoms as they may be due to an outflow obstruction.

6. Day care

   An assessment of the general state of health ASA 1, 2 or stable 3. Instructions: No food from the night before, drinks up to two hours before surgery. Distance from hospital and transport arrangements. Someone to accompany them home and to stay with them for 24 hours. What are the home circumstances, is there a phone at home? Not to drive a car, return to work or do anything that might be affected by the recent drug administration which could affect their judgement for 24 hours. This could include signing a legal document, operating machinery including cooking. Do they know the arrangements for seeking help, pain relief at home and follow up?

7. Smoker, alcohol intake, other drugs and allergies, teeth, past history and previous anaesthetics, other symptoms.

Answers – FOLLOW ON STATION 1

1. **False** – If there are no renal symptoms and the bladder symptoms are recent it is unlikely.

2. **True** – A gastrectomy could remove intrinsic factor and cause pernicious anaemia.

3. **False** – There is no evidence that a haemoglobin of 9 g/dl is associated with an increased morbidity. Transfusion might be relevant as part of the resuscitation for hypovolaemia and acute blood loss, but not in the first instance for anaemia or a routine cystoscopy. It is more important to diagnose a cause of the anaemia.

4. **True** – This is the commonest source of infection in some countries.

5. **False**

6. **True**

7. **False** – The usual cause of a raised creatinine is impaired renal function.

8. **False** – No change in BP but a rise in heart rate would be expected.

9. **True** – Also associated with rheumatoid arthritis.

10. **False** – A reduced glomerular filtration rate (GFR) may reduce urine volume but failure of tubular reabsorption (which usually accompanies glomerular dysfunction) may lead to a high urine output.

Answers – HISTORY 2

Scenario: You are an elderly lady with post menopausal bleeding and atrial fibrillation. Hypertensive taking an ACE inhibitor, low dose aspirin and warfarin. You are suffering from "fainting attacks", which have become less frequent since starting the warfarin.

This case illustrates the range of problems, that the elderly may suffer from. Also the range of drug interactions in the elderly.

1. The reason for the hysterectomy. Problems of the elderly – particularly general health, exercise tolerance and drugs.

2. The causes of bleeding:
   • Carcinoma - weight loss.
   • Clotting disorder.
   • Anticoagulant therapy.
   • Leukaemia or other marrow dysfunction - bruising.

   How much blood has been lost and when did the symptom start?

   The effect of blood loss: is the patient anaemic with CVS symptoms of breathlessness, angina, oedema and limited exercise tolerance?

3. Ask about the amount of blood loss and for how long – any clots? Ask about general symptoms and particularly in the elderly about drug history. Symptoms of weakness, syncope or transient ischaemic episodes, angina, breathlessness and orthopnea, oedema, exercise limit.

4. It might be logical to link the ACE inhibitor to falls in blood pressure causing syncope if the two started at the same time or if the patient also uses a diuretic. A diuretic such as frusemide causes loss of salt and water. This may lead to thirst, increased water intake, a low serum sodium and aldosterone production. If an ACE inhibitor is added at this stage there is an increased diuresis and a possible fall in blood pressure.

   First think of other causes of syncope:

   Heart block, anaemia, hypoglycaemia, arteriosclerosis of carotid arteries, other drugs.

   Ask about the possible side effects of ACE inhibitors: Dose, duration of administration. Have there been other treatments for hypertension such as diuretics; ACE inhibitors are used when thiazide diuretics and beta blockers are contraindicated and are particularly indicated in insulin-dependant diabetics. It may be relevant to consider whether the ACE inhibitor was used due to an adverse reaction to another anti-hypertensive drug and what that reaction was.

Did the diuretics aggravate the patient's diabetes or gout or beta blockers aggravate asthma? If a condition like hypertension is mentioned consider the effect it may be having on other organs such as kidneys, eyes, and the vessels of heart and brain.

5. Low dose aspirin 75 mg daily is taken as an antithrombotic agent to delay arteriosclerosis in angina or to reduce emboli causing TIAs. Larger doses of 600 mg 6 hourly are used for anti- inflammatory pain relief. In this case check on coagulation status, renal function with ACE inhibitors and aspirin and possible link to nasal polyps and asthma.

6. Warfarin is probably given for DVT or atrial fibrillation (caused by the hypertension) with evidence of emboli. Has she had either diagnosed? It might be aggravating the blood loss.

7. Teeth, allergies, smoker, alcohol.

Answers – FOLLOW ON STATION 2

1. Full blood count. May show iron deficiency anaemia implying chronic anaemia. Remember that as people get older their haemoglobin falls. By 80 years old 10g/100ml can be normal.

2. Renal function tests: creatinine clearance falls with age, NSAIDs may reduce renal function and lead to salt and water retention, hypertension may reduce renal function. ACE inhibitors may aggravate existing renal-vascular disease. Diuretics will reduce serum sodium and potassium concentrations by their renal action. This effect is aggravated by thirst which leads to increased water intake and a further dilution of serum electrolytes.

3. ECG. Look for evidence of ischaemia, ventricular hypertrophy, previous infarction or dysrhythmias, heart block.

4. Prothrombin time (normal 12-15 seconds): extended to x 2 to x 3 depending on the reason for the prescription of warfarin.

5. CXR. To assess size of heart, exclude carcinoma – a primary tumour if smoking – secondaries from pelvis not common, but ovarian tumours can be associated with pleural effusions.

6. Convert to heparin. Stop warfarin at least 48 hours preoperatively. Aim to get the Activated Partial Thromboplastin Time (normal 30-45 seconds) with heparin to x 1.5 to x 2.5 control.

7. Four from:.

   Anaemia due to blood loss.

   Transient ischaemic episodes giving weakness or blindness due to arteriosclerosis of emboli from atrial fibrillation

   Atrial fibrillation with emboli.

   Heart block and other cardiac dysrhythmias giving syncope.

   Hypoglycaemia.

   Blindness.

   Foot drop from sacral root compression and weakness
   linked to a lumbar spine problem.

   Neuromuscular diseases like MS or motor neurone disease.

8. No. It is important to be aware of the cause of a low haemoglobin concentration. 10 g/100 ml is normal for elderly people. The operation may not be associated with a large blood loss and providing the patient has a proper diet they will restore their haemoglobin post-operatively. It is important to maintain circulating blood volume but there is no evidence that a haemoglobin of 8 g or 9 g/100 ml leads to a worse outcome than those at 12 g/100 ml. There are

compensations for a low PCV; reduced viscosity, and a shift in the oxygen dissociation curve to the right due to a rise in 2,3-DPG, when the haemoglobin has fallen over a period of time.

9. Oxygen flux is Haemoglobin concentration x 1.34 ml/g x arterial oxygen saturation x cardiac output.

So Hb 150 g/l x 1.34 x 5 l/min = 1000ml/minute of oxygen. Basal demand 250ml/minute.

Hb 80 g/l x 1.34 x 5 l/minute = 536 ml/minute. Compensation can occur by increasing heart rate and/or stroke volume.

Answers – HISTORY 3

Scenario: You are a patient with a thyroid swelling, clinically thyrotoxic. Breathless on exertion, atrial fibrillation, on warfarin and aspirin.

1. Start with an introduction and proceed to ask about the present complaint. How long has it been present, when first noticed? Decide if the patient has a mass which is enlarging; and then symptoms suggesting a thyrotoxic, hypothyroid or euthyroid state.

2. Neck swelling. Are their symptoms of pressure on the airway?

   This is the upper airway so stridor implies tracheal narrowing. Infiltration into the surrounding tissue may occur with cancer, not a goitre. Hoarseness by pressure on the recurrent laryngeal nerve implies carcinoma of the thyroid.

   Hyperthyroid symptoms: hyperactivity, sweating, palpitations particularly in the elderly, loss of weight with increased appetite, diarrhoea and heat intolerance. Signs of tremor, warm peripheries, pretibial oedema and exophthalmos. Alterations in menstruation.

   Hypothyroid symptoms: weight gain, dry thin hair and hair loss, gruff or deep toned voice, constipation, cold intolerance and a slowing of mental activity. Bradycardia and pericardial effusions may give rise to breathlessness.

3. The patient may be taking carbimazole. Carbimazole is commonly used to inhibit the formation of thyroid hormones. Be sure there are no side effects: nausea, rashes, pruritus, jaundice and rarely life threatening blood dyscrasia presenting as a sore throat. Propylthiouracil is used when there are side effects to carbimazole. Propranolol may be used for supraventricular tachycardias associated with hyperthyroid states.

   About 5 days before surgery iodine is given to reduce the vascularity of the gland.

4. There is a link between hyperthyroidism and other autoimmune conditions such as pernicious anaemia and myasthenia gravis. Symptoms of muscle weakness and lid lag. Anaemia might give CVS symptoms and fatigue. Where does the patient come from? Goitres are more common in mountainous areas where iodine is deficient in the water.

5. There might be: palpitations from atrial fibrillation, a thyrotoxic crisis, a myocardial infarction or conditions unrelated to the thyrotoxicosis, such as a chest infection, pulmonary embolism, oesophagitis, or herpes zoster. Check that this was chest pain and not an abdominal pain.

   It is important to ask about possible complications of a myocardial infarction such as: angina, palpitations, breathlessness and oedema.

   Drugs: Aspirin 75mg or more daily, beta blocker, GTN, anticoagulants, calcium channel blocker.

6. Previous anaesthetics, smoking, alcohol, other drugs and allergies, teeth, veins and family history.

Answers – FOLLOW ON STATION 3

1. Full blood count. Both hypo- and hyper-thyroidism can be associated with pernicious anaemia (also with myasthenia gravis).

2. ECG - Hyperthyroidism is associated with atrial fibrillation.

3. Neck: Imaging –CT scan or MRI scan if there is a large or retrosternal thyroid. Indirect laryngoscopy for cord movement. A lung scan if concerned about emboli.

4. Free T4 low and TSH high in hypothyroidism. TSH low if pituitary disease. In hyperthyroidism the TSH will be suppressed and the T3 or T4 raised (normal T4 60-160nmol/l). Microsomal and thyroglobin antibodies are present in most cases of thyrotoxicosis.

5. In anxiety the resting pulse will fall during sleep, but remain raised in thyrotoxicosis. The periphery is warm in thyrotoxicosis and cold in anxiety.

6. The corneas of the eyes, particularly with exophthalmos.

7. Inhibits cyclo-oxygenase in platelets. This reduces the production of TXA2 which is a vasoconstrictor and initiates the platelet release reaction leading to a platelet plug.

8. Blocks cyclo-oxygenase function:
   - peptic ulceration and gastrointestinal bleeding,
   - impaired renal function with salt and water retention,
   - reduced blood coagulability due to reduced platelet aggregation,
   - bronchospasm in susceptible adults with nasal polyps,
   - altered liver enzymes.

9. Immediate: haemorrhage, lesions of the recurrent laryngeal nerve, tracheal malacia; all can cause respiratory obstruction. Thyrotoxic crisis.

10. Days or weeks: hypoparathyroidism (<1%) but short term tetany in 10%. Longer term: hypothyroidism (<10%) and hyperthyroidism (<5%).

Answers – HISTORY 4

Scenario: You are a patient with bronchiectasis (but would not tell the examining doctor this diagnosis unless specifically asked: "Do you have Bronchiectasis?"). You are working and reasonably active. For arthroscopy as a day patient. Wheeze, sputum, bronchodilators. Measles as a child and several periods in hospital in teens with postural drainage. You had a lobectomy 10 years ago.

1. Two issues to start with:

   a. Why the arthroscopy? What is the problem - e.g. pain? How long has it been a problem, what caused it?

   b. General health – what are the main symptoms; drugs, past history and operations, social history?

   Five minutes goes very quickly so do not get fixed or dwell on just one problem. At this stage you know the reason for the operation and at least one symptom.

2. Ask about the chest symptoms in a systematic way, otherwise you may jump to the wrong diagnosis.

   • Cough, is it productive?

   • Sputum colour and how much? Chronic bronchitis is a cough productive of sputum for more than 3 months of the year and for more than 2 years in succession.

   • Haemoptysis - could be chronic bronchitis, carcinoma, or tuberculosis.

   • Wheeze. When is it worse – morning or evening; what aggravates it – allergies; any hospital admissions?

   • Shortness of breath at rest or on exercise. How much is the exercise tolerance? Wheeze and breathlessness are symptoms of respiratory and cardiovascular diseases.

   • Pain.

   How long have the symptoms been a problem. Does the patient have an acute or chronic problem?

   Differential diagnosis:

Acute	– pneumonia, pneumothorax (unlikely in an examination).
Chronic	– bronchitis, bronchiectasis, asthma, restrictive disease following injury, gassing or fractures, occupational disease following mining, carcinoma. Sarcoidosis affects women with fatigue and weight loss; tuberculosis may induce night sweats, haemoptysis and weight loss.

   Haemoptysis – think carcinoma, bronchitis, TB, bronchiectasis, coagulation disorder, left ventricular failure if frothy.

   The inhalers may be salbutamol or a steroid. Is the patient (or have they been) taking systemic steroids?

3. Childhood symptoms suggest a congenital problem or childhood illness, trauma. Cystic fibrosis. Bronchiectasis following a childhood pneumonia may follow illness such as measles or whooping cough, or an inhaled foreign body – peanut, childhood asthma.

Ask about: Treatment with antibiotics, steroids and bronchodilators. Bronchodilators are used for conditions other than asthma. Postural drainage. Operations to remove part of the lung which is diseased. Treatment for tuberculosis or sarcoidosis.

4. Breathlessness can be respiratory or cardiovascular in origin. Breathless upright or with exercise implies limited gaseous exchange either due to reduced cardiac or respiratory function.

Respiratory breathlessness – ask about "wheeze" rather than asthma which is one specific type of wheeze. Alveolar and small airway obstruction will first cause an expiratory wheeze. Upper airway obstruction first gives an inspiratory wheeze. Asthma is associated with reversible airway obstruction which varies in severity during the day, usually worse in the morning. Chronic obstructive airways disease gives rise to a non reversible wheeze.

Cardiovascular breathlessness due to congestion in the lung with oedema will get worse with lying down suggesting: orthopnoea, or paroxysmal nocturnal dyspnoea (PND). PND suggests pulmonary oedema but can be asthma. The wheeze of pulmonary oedema is more permanent than a respiratory wheeze, may be relieved by diuretics and failure will give frothy sputum.

While talking you may notice signs of breathlessness, cyanosis, hand tremor, and clubbing, but it is not part of your task to examine the patient in the history taking station.

5. Miners, or workers with asbestos or in a dusty atmosphere can develop restrictive lung diseases, including asbestosis. Farmers working in damp barns get farmer's lung.

Hobbies: keeping pigeons can cause an allergic alveolitis.

Smoker and lung cancer.

6. In a person with a chest complaint consider: smoking, do they take regular antibiotics, do they get influenza immunisation in the winter? You would not want to operate in the winter. Have they required hospital admission and ventilator support?

General health, Teeth, Alcohol intake.

Answers – FOLLOW ON STATION 4

1-3. Full blood count for polycythaemia. Lung function tests: Vitalograph and check for reversibility with a bronchodilator; arterial gases if respiratory failure is suspected; diffusion assessment with carbon monoxide transfer factor; CXR to eliminate carcinoma, assess presence of dilated bronchi, thick walls and cysts, extent of infection and size of heart; Sputum for culture; ECG signs of right heart strain and right ventricular hypertrophy – right axis deviation, inverted T waves in V1–V5 and tall P wave of p pulmonale.

4. False – The patient needs a broad spectrum antibiotic.

5. An obstructive airway disease.

6. A bronchodilator – a beta$_2$ stimulant, possibly steroids.

7. Exclude a tuberculosis infection, or carcinoma. Consider a fibre optic bronchoscopy and biopsy, sputum for cytology or staining with Ziehl-Nielson stain.

8, 9. Pain relief, oxygen, bronchodilators, possibly steroids, chest physiotherapy with postural drainage and humidification to make coughing easier and effective. Retained secretions may be a major problem.

10. If possible give the normal oral medication. Inhaled steroids may be sufficient. Consider increasing the steroid dose by giving hydrocortisone 50mg or 100mg before or during surgery and 6 hourly for 24 hours. Additional therapy will depend on the nature of the surgery and the control of the condition for which the steroids are being given.

Answers – HISTORY 5

Scenario: Arthritis – lead to diagnosis of rheumatoid rather than osteoarthritis. Operation: cholecystectomy for abdominal pain, might not be gall stones. Diabetic on oral hypoglycaemic and diet.

1. Take your lead from the introductory statement. The type of arthritis and the symptoms leading to the cholecystectomy. How long has the patient had symptoms, when did they start?

2. Osteoarthritis, rheumatoid arthritis, ankylosing spondylitis or linked to psoriasis, polymyalgia rheumatica, gout, or a connective tissue disorder?

   Ask about duration of illness and possible injury. Types of joints affected. Pain, type, when worse and what makes it easier.

   Osteoarthritis pain is in the knees, hips, hands, aggravated by movement, eased by rest, morning stiffness, large joint deformity. Osteoarthritis often affects a single joint and may follow a traumatic insult.

   Rheumatoid arthritis causes pain in the small joints of hands and feet, with morning stiffness but improving with activity. About 25% of patients have only one joint affected, general fatigue and malaise common, other organs affected. Non weight bearing joints are more involved with RA which is usually a polyarthropathy affecting joints in a symmetrical pattern.

   Osteo- and rheumatoid-arthritis are both familial. Single joint involvement in gout.

3. Neck movement. Atlanto-axial subluxation can give rise to serious neurological signs. Mouth opening may be limited by temperomandibular joint limitation of movement. Renal function anaemia, lung function.

   Anaemia is common. Thrombocytosis is linked to the activity of the disease. Lungs: pleural effusions, and small airway disease. The skin can be affected by a vasculitis which leads to ischaemia and gangrene of fingers and toes.

   Possible arteritis with rheumatoid and autoimmune diseases may involve: kidneys, respiratory or cardiovascular systems giving breathlessness. Sight is affected in Sjögren's syndrome – dry eyes or scleritis in RA and auto-immune disease, steroid effect or psoriasis.

4. Analgesics, RA specific agents and steroids and for how long? Steroids may need supplementation around the time of operation. Steroid effects: on skin and subcutaneous tissue, hypertension, diabetic state, osteoporotic fractures, mental effect paranoia or depression, proximal muscle wasting, peptic ulceration exacerbation. NSAIDs. Agents to suppress the disease process such as Gold Penicillamine, Azothioprine.

5. Differentiate pain above the diaphragm: myocardial infarction, pneumonia, hiatus hernia; below the diaphragm: cholecystitis, peptic ulcer, diabetes, porphyria, bowel disorders such as irritable bowel syndrome, inflammatory bowel disease. Has the patient been jaundiced?

6. Diabetes. Diet and drugs - which ones and for how long? How well controlled is the diabetes? Urine or blood sampling; at home or special clinic, role of diabetic specialist nurse. Diabetes affects many organs. Ask about: features of arteriosclerosis, angina, transient ischaemic episodes, angina, claudication. Renal function – kidney infection and glomerular impairment and vascular changes similar to hypertensive changes.

Neurological changes will affect 80% of diabetics. The legs may be affected by a sensory or autonomic neuropathy leading to postural hypotension causing syncope on standing. Autonomic neuropathy is common affecting the bladder function and incontinence. Ask about paraesthesia, numbness or burning sensations, diarrhoea.

Eye sight is affected by cataracts and new vessels growing on to the iris and retina, and a sixth nerve palsy.

Weight loss.

The foot is at risk from ischaemia, ulcers and infection. Leg pain and ischaemia may limit exercise making it difficult to assess the severity of cardiovascular or respiratory disease.

Arterial occlusion symptoms may also be present as angina, claudication or stroke.

Answers – FOLLOW ON STATION 5

1 to 4.
- CXR for heart size, pains above diaphragm — pneumonia, pneumothorax, hiatus hernia.
- ECG for ischaemia.
- Full blood count for anaemia or infection.
- – Creatinine urea and electrolytes for renal function.
  - Liver function tests if jaundiced.
  - Glucose and glycosolated haemoglobin to indicate current and recent diabetic control.
- X-ray neck in extension and flexion for atlanto — axial stability in rheumatoid arthritis.

5. The patient should receive vitamin K pre-operatively, and mannitol or frusemide before, during or after the operation.

6. True

7. False – Normochromic and normocytic.

8. False – Insulin with glucose pre-operatively and potassium, depending on serum levels.

9. False – Every hour.

10. True – Through an opening in the diaphragm such as a hernia or a defect left from previous surgery.

The issues raised by this case are: Differentiation of the common types of arthritis. The importance of recognising the multi-organ involvement of rheumatoid arthritis. A jaundiced patient may have clotting and renal impairment. A diabetic should be converted to an insulin regime which must include simultaneous glucose and potassium. Consider the effects of laparoscopy.

SKILL

3

SKILL 1

(Answers on page 59)

Try to complete all the questions. Have a guess if there is no negative marking on this station. You might come back to a question at the end if there is time.

You are asked to demonstrate how to assess a patient's airway.

Questions

1. – Write down, in order, the features that you will check.

2. – What might inspection show?

3. – How far should the mouth open? What may limit opening?

4. – The neck will normally move freely. Which condition may be associated with good movement but is a dangerous situation during intubation?

5. – How can the shortness of the neck be assessed?

6. – What is the Mallampati score? Describe exactly the grades.

7. – What is the relationship between the Mallampati score and the Cormack and Lehane score?

8. – Describe all the grades of the Cormack and Lehane score.

9. – What is the significance of a history of snoring?

SKILL 2

(Answers on page 60)

You are asked to demonstrate the technique of cricothyroid puncture on a neck manikin.

Questions

1. Demonstrate the correct position for the head.

2. Where is the needle introduced?

3. If oxygen is infused through a cannula without ventilating the lungs what will happen to the arterial carbon dioxide level?

4. Name at least two possible complications associated with cricothyroid puncture.

5. Is a percutaneous tracheostomy performed at the same site?

6. Name three indications for cricothyroid puncture.

7. At what depth will the cricothyroid membrane be punctured?

8. How would you deal with an obstruction to expiration once cricothyroid ventilation has been established?

9. Name one contraindication to cricothyroid puncture?

10. Label the anatomical structures on the diagram (opposite).

SAGITTAL SECTION OF THE NECK
(LABEL THE STRUCTURES MARKED ON THE DIAGRAM)

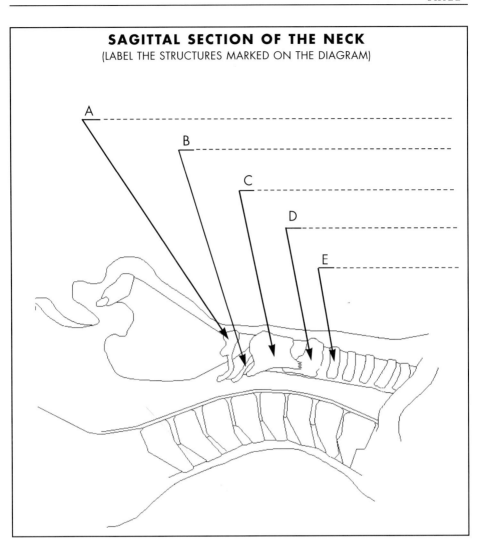

A _____

B _____

C _____

D _____

E _____

SKILL 3

(Answers on page 61)

You are asked to demonstrate cricoid pressure on a manikin of the neck.

Questions

1. – On the diagram opposite draw in the position of:
    - The thyroid cartilage.
    - The hyoid bone.
    - The trachea.
    - The internal jugular vein.
    - Sternomastoid and recurrent laryngeal nerves.

2. – Which cartilage is pressure applied to?

3. – What is the cartilage pressed against?

4. – Which fingers are used?

5. – How are the hands placed?

6. – When should the pressure be removed?

7. – When will this manoeuvre be less effective?

8. – Who was Sellick?

9. – What amount of pressure should be used?

10. – What is the minimum time for satisfactory pre-oxygenation?

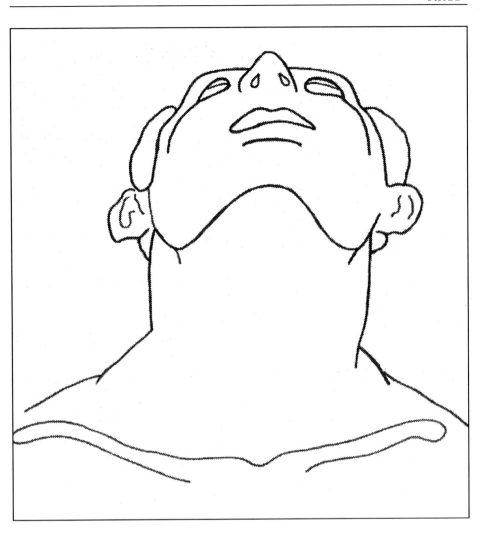

SKILL 4

(*Answers on page 62*)

The diagram below includes a number of errors.

Questions

1. – How many can you spot?

2. – Draw lines to connect the apparatus to ensure a negative pressure on the drain of not more than 5 cmH$_2$O.

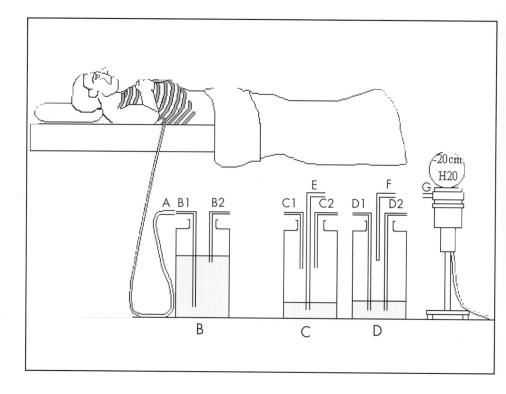

SKILL 5

(Answers on page 63)

The diagram below includes a number of errors.

Questions

1. – How many can you spot?

2. – Is the pressure trace correct?

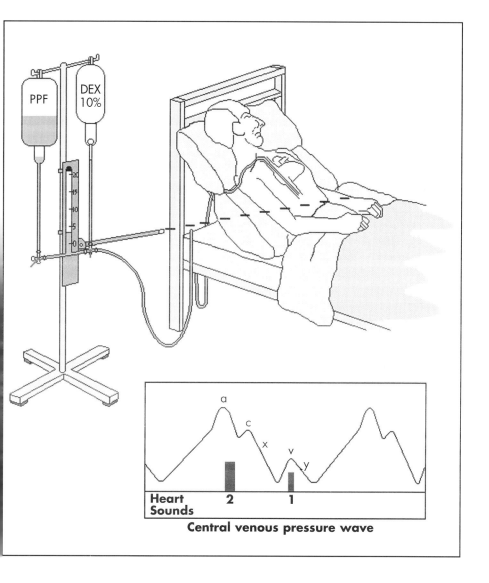

Central venous pressure wave

SKILL 6

(Answers on page 64)

The diagram below includes a number of errors.

Question

1. – How many can you spot?

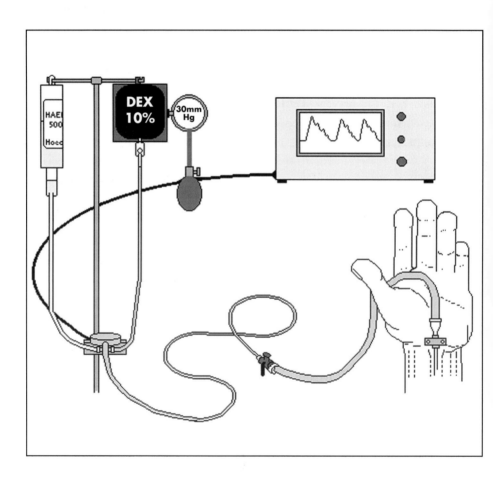

SKILL 7

(Answers on page 65)

Three-in-one-block

Question

1. – Label the diagram of the inguinal region below. Describe the landmarks for identifying the point for injection to achieve a three-in-one block.

2. – Which nerves should be blocked in performing a three-in-one block?

3. – Which nerve roots do these nerves come from?

4. – Name at least two situations for which three in one block might be relevant.

5. – What volume of local anaesthetic is used?

6. – What precautions are taken during injection of the local anaesthetic?

7. – When using a nerve stimulator to locate the nerve:

   a. What current is supplied by the stimulator?

   b. Which are stimulated first as the current is increased, motor or sensory nerves?

   c. What current should be used so that the stimulus is not painful when applied directly to the nerve?

   d. Which pole of the stimulator should be applied to the nerve and which to the skin?

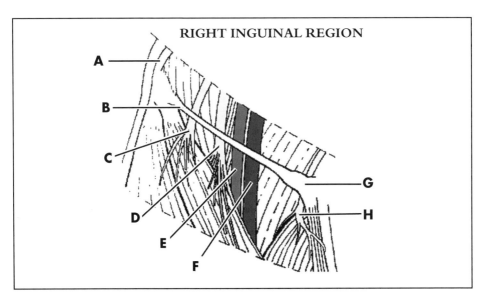

RIGHT INGUINAL REGION

A
B
C
D
E
F
G
H

SKILL 8

(Answers on page 66)

Questions

1. – Label the structures marked on the sagittal section of the spine shown opposite.

2. – In the adult the spinal cord ends at the level of lumbar 3. True False

3. – In adults the subarachnoid space ends at the level of lumbar 4. True False

4. – The epidural space can be detected by using loss of resistance to air. True False

5. – The depth from skin to epidural space is an average of about 4cm. True False

6. – The depth from skin to epidural space is further when the paramedian approach is used than when the midline approach is used. True False

7. – The average total volume of each epidural space is 2cc. True False

8. – A test dose of 2cc local anaesthetic at L2 will give a sensory blockade of the thighs if placed into the CSF. True False

9. – The Tuohy needle is so named because it has a blunt end. True False

10. – There is no epidural space inside the skull. True False

11. – An epidural can be performed through the sacral hiatus. True False

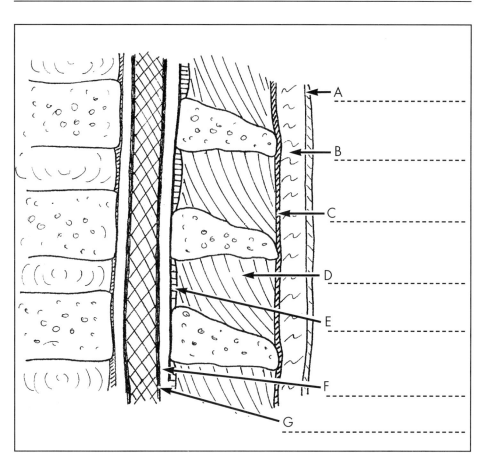

A ------------------------

B ------------------------

C ------------------------

D ------------------------

E ------------------------

F ------------------------

G ------------------------

SKILL 9

(Answers on page 67)

Local anaesthetic blocks for eye surgery.

Questions

1. – What position should the eye be in for a periorbital nerve block and which position should be avoided?

2. – Describe the first stage in the application of local anaesthetic.

3. – What is the point of entry of the needle for a periorbital block?

4. – How does a periorbital block differ from a retrobulbar block?

5. – What is the furthest distance a needle should be introduced for a periorbital block?

6. – Which muscle is supplied by the seventh cranial nerve and is blocked for eye surgery?

7. – Name two complications of a periorbital block.

8. – How would you diagnose and treat a retrobulbar haematoma?

9. – Apart from 2% lignocaine and 0.75% bupivacaine what else might be included in a solution for periorbital block and why?

10. – What are the features of a successful periorbital block?

ANSWERS
SKILL

1, 2. General inspection. Visual appearance: obesity, facial scaring or deformity, cervical and thoracic spinal deformity, neck short or limited movement, mouth opening – prominent mandible or upper incisors.

Specific diseases: Rheumatoid arthritis, thoracic kyphosis, burns of the head and neck, congenital abnormality of head and neck.

3. Mouth opening: ask the patient to open their mouth. Can three or more fingers be inserted in the sagittal plane? Is movement of the tempero-mandibular joint limited?

4. Neck movement. Extension and flexion. A normal head should extend on the neck to at least 45° to the horizontal. Reduced movement may result from osteoarthritis, ankylosing spondylosis, rheumatoid arthritis and previous surgery. In rheumatoid arthritis an X-ray in extension and flexion for evidence of movement at the atlanto-occipital joint is essential to exclude subluxation.

5. Short neck: measure the thyro-mental distance with the head extended. Under 6 cm, or three finger widths, may be a problem for intubation.

6. Mallampati score.

Open the mouth and see the tonsillar fauces and pillars *score 1*. The uvula and upper fauces *score 2*. The soft palate and base of uvula *score 3*. The hard palate only (no soft palate visible) *score 4*. 3 and 4 may be a difficult intubation.

7. There is a correlation, but not an absolute one, between the two scores.

8. The score is: Total larynx seen *1*. Only the posterior larynx seen *2*. Epiglottis but no arytenoids seen *3*. No epiglottis seen *4*.

9. Snoring indicates a narrowing of some point in the airway when the muscles relax that support the airway between the sternum and the mandible. One site for obstruction is the tongue vibrating against the posterior pharyngeal wall or inlet to the larynx. This suggests there will be a poor view of the larynx at laryngoscopy due to the tongue or epiglottis blocking the view of the larynx. The patient will also be more prone to airway obstruction postoperatively.

Answers – SKILL 2

1. The patient is supine with the neck extended.

2. The cricothyroid membrane - which connects the thyroid cartilage to the cricoid cartilage – is punctured anteriorly, in the mid line.

3. Arterial carbon dioxide will rise at the rate of 0.5 kPa (3 mmHg) every minute.

4. Complications include: puncturing the carotid artery, internal jugular vein, perforation of the oesophagus, pretracheal inflation of gas, barotrauma to the trachea, surgical emphysema in the neck as gas leaks back around the catheter puncture site, bronchial rupture and pneumothorax.

5. No. It involves puncturing the space between the first and second tracheal rings.

6. *a*. Emergency control of the airway.

   b. Topical anaesthesia of the larynx e.g. for laryngospasm.

   c. Retrograde intubation of the larynx.

   d. Jet ventilation for laryngoscopy.

   e. Clearance of secretions following surgery, particularly thoracic surgery.

7. About 0.5 inches or 1 cm.

8. Try to relieve the obstruction by an oral airway, mouth suction or forward traction on the jaw. A second catheter may need to be introduced.

9. Trauma to the throat making it difficult to locate the landmarks. A large thyroid goitre or tumour obscuring the larynx.

10. A – Hyoid

    B – Epiglottis cartilage

    C – Thyroid cartilage

    D – Cricoid cartilage

    E – Trachea and trachea ring.

Answers – SKILL 3

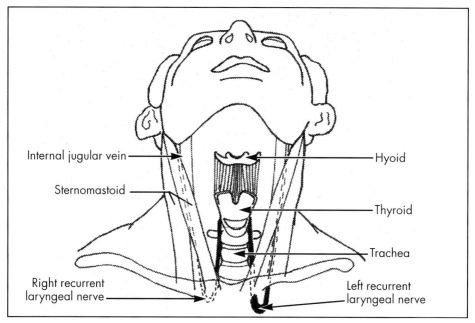

Internal jugular vein
Sternomastoid
Right recurrent laryngeal nerve
Hyoid
Thyroid
Trachea
Left recurrent laryngeal nerve

1. As above.

2. The cricoid cartilage.

3. The body of the 6th cervical vertebra.

4. The thumb and middle finger are pressed onto the cartilage while the index finger is used to steady the mid-line.

5. One hand is used to press the cricoid cartilage while the other is placed behind the cervical spine. This is a bimanual manoeuvre.

6. Pressure is removed once the assistant has inflated the cuff or if the patient starts to vomit forcibly, to prevent rupture of the oesophagus.

7. In the presence of a nasogastric tube, a laryngeal mask and an oesophageal pouch. Once a laryngeal mask is in place it may be possible to apply cricoid pressure with effect but the presence of cricoid pressure may prevent the placement of the laryngeal mask.

8. A London anaesthetist who described the technique in the 1960's.

9. Up to 44 Newtons. This is equivalent to four 1 kg bags of sugar.

10. Adequate pre-oxygenation will occur in about 6 deep breaths which will replace the nitrogen in the lungs. It takes a further 3 minutes to replace most of the rest of the nitrogen in the rest of the body.

Answers – SKILL 4

1. Wrong site to insert a catheter into the chest. Either 2nd space mid clavicular line or 4/5th space mid axillary line.

   Connecting tubing too long and draping on floor. Likely to increase the possibility of disconnection, kinking and the introduction of infection.

   The drainage bottles B,C, and D have no stoppers in the tops.

   The water depth in bottle B is too high, increasing the resistance to expanding the lung.

   The drainage tube B1 is too far into the water. This will increase the expiratory pressure and the pneumothorax may not expand.

   B2 should not be under the water.

   Bottle D is wrongly made up, C is correct. In D the tubes at the side are wrongly under the water while the centre tube is in free air. This will not produce a negative pressure.

2. To obtain about 5 cmH$_2$O – pipe B2 is connected to C1, then C2 connected to G and the suction turned on. The negative pressure is controlled by the depth of E under the water.

Answers – SKILL 5

1. Wrong agents in the infusion bags. The solution used to make a reading should be normal saline, or Hartman's solution. 5% dextrose if there is concern about the conduction of an electric current.

   One administration set has no ball valve in the reservoir.

   One administration set reservoir is empty of fluid.

   No controllers on giving sets.

   No tap at bottom of measuring column.

   Sealed top to measuring column.

   Connecting tubing too long and draping on floor. Likely to cause damping and will increase possibility of disconnection, kinking and introducing infection.

   Catheter tip in inferior vena cava and not at entry to right atrium.

   The reading as drawn is below zero and is not physiologically possible, unless the patient breathes in against a resistance to create a marked negative intra-thoracic pressure. The reading is not compatible with a venous return sustaining a cardiac output. The patient should ideally be flat if an accurate reading is being made.

2. The a,c,v trace relating to the heart sounds is not correctly labelled. The a wave should be lined up with the first heart sound. The second heart sound occurs with the v wave.

Answers – SKILL 6

1. The fluids for infusion are wrong. There should only be one isotonic crystalloid, such as saline, to infuse into the artery.

   The pressure in the surrounding bag is too low. It should be at least 50% above systolic pressure. There is no pressure bag on the gelatin line which runs directly to the arterial line.

   There is no clamp on the giving sets.

   There is no fluid in one of the reservoir chambers.

   There is no ball valve in one chamber.

   The tubing between the transducer and the patient is too long, and too wide.

   There is no tap near to the patient from which to sample arterial blood or to flush the line.

   There is no obvious continuous flushing device.

   The pressure trace is resonant.

   The cannula should enter the wrist between abductor pollucis longus and flexor carpi radialis (FCR). Not FCR and palmaris longus.

Answers – SKILL 7

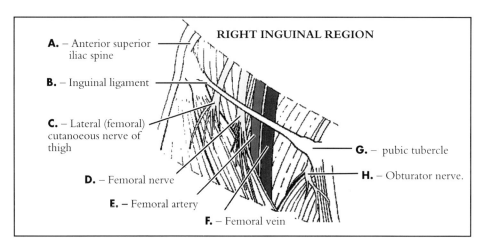

A. – Anterior superior iliac spine

B. – Inguinal ligament

C. – Lateral (femoral) cutanoeous nerve of thigh

D. – Femoral nerve

E. – Femoral artery

F. – Femoral vein

RIGHT INGUINAL REGION

G. – pubic tubercle

H. – Obturator nerve.

1. A-H as above

   Palpate the anterior superior iliac spine and the pubic tubercle. Mark the inguinal ligament which joins these two points. Mark the mid point of this line which should be the point at which the femoral artery can be felt pulsating. The femoral nerve lies about 1 cm or a fingers width lateral to the artery. A short bevelled needle is introduced over the nerve and below the inguinal ligament. Pulsation of the artery may be felt as the needle in advanced. Paraesthesia will be obtained when the needle is near the nerve at a depth of about 3-4 cm.

2. Femoral, lateral (femoral) cutaneous nerve of the thigh and obturator nerves.

3. The anterior primary rami of lumbar 2,3 and 4 which form the lumbar plexus.

4. Pain relief following operations on the knee, shaft and neck of femur, skin grafts from the thigh.

5. 20 ml was originally recommended and is suitable for a femoral block. 30 ml is used for a 3 in 1 block.

6. Monitor for intravascular injection. Apply pressure over the femoral nerve distal to the point of injection to encourage proximal spread of the local anaesthetic.

7. *a.* 6-8 volts limited to 30 milliamps. The impulse is 0.3 millisecond or less duration at 2Hz or 50Hz.

   b. Motor nerves are stimulated first at 2Hz. Sensory nerves are stimulated at 50Hz. High frequencies (50Hz) produce pain before lower frequencies (2Hz).

   c. 2Hz or 50Hz and under 0.5 milliamp.

   d. The negative is applied to the nerve as there is a greater density of current around the negative and so about 30% less current is required to produce a stimulus. It also helps to localise the nerve more accurately.

Answers – SKILL 8

1. A – skin
    B – subcutaneous tissue
    C – supraspinous ligament
    D – interspinous ligament
    E – ligamentum flavum
    F – epidural space
    G – dura mater.

2. **False** The subarachnoid space extends to the sacrum in the foetus. Due to the bone growing faster than the nerve tissue of the cord the cord finishes at about lumbar 1 in the adult.

3. **False** The subarachnoid finishes at sacral 1, below which the dura continues as filum terminale

4. **True** The space can be detected by loss of resistance to air or fluid, or the negative pressure in the lumbar region.

5. **True** The normal range is 3 to 5 cm.

6. **True**

7. **False** The average volume is 4 cc; greater in the sacral region. The space is occupied by nerve roots, vessels and adipose tissue, so this is not the volume of local anaesthetic required to fill the space.

8. **True** The thigh is innervated by L1,2,3 nerve roots.

9. **False** The blunt end is the Huber point. The side opening is the Tuohy needle.

10. **True** The epidural space ends at the foramen magnum and is only a potential space inside the skull.

11. **True** The sacral hiatus is where the spine of S5 might have been and is a portal into the sacral canal.

1. The patient should look straight ahead. In the past the patient might have looked up and medially for a retrobulbar block. This brings the optic nerve and vessels into prominence and into a position where they are more likely to be punctured.

2. The conjunctiva and cornea are anaesthetized with 4% lignocaine, amethocaine 0.5% or oxybuprocaine 0.4% eye drops. Cocaine is avoided as it may damage the cornea. In order to reduce patient discomfort a series of instillations are made starting with a dilute solution.

3. At the inferior-lateral angle of the eye through the conjunctiva. A second point may be used: through the conjunctiva between the superior orbital notch and the medial canthus.

4. *a.* The retrobulbar block needle is usually introduced through the skin of the eyelid and pierces the muscle cone.

   b. The periorbital block needle enters through the conjunctiva and stays outside the muscle cone.

5. 25 mm.

6. The orbicularis oculi is blocked to prevent involuntary blinking. If the seventh nerve is not blocked in the orbit a separate block can be made. Part of the nerve can be blocked outside the lateral margin of the orbit in the temporal area or all the nerve is blocked in front of the tragus in the parotid area.

7. Vasovagal reaction, haematoma, total spinal with local anaesthetic entering the CSF and intravascular reactions to local anaesthetic.

8. The eye becomes tense and pushes forward. Apply pressure for 20 to 30 minutes, delay surgery and possibly perform a canthotomy.

9. Hyalase 5 units/ml to encourage spread of the local anaesthetic and possibly reduce intra ocular pressure. Adrenaline or other vasoconstrictor to reduce bleeding and prolong the effect of the block and orbital akinesia.

10. Anaesthesia of the eye, a dilated pupil, exophthalmos, reduced intra ocular pressure and an immobile eye.

PHYSICAL EXAMINATION

4

We consider that there are at least two aspects to physical examination: the examination and making deductions from the findings. You must have a method and practice performing a routine examination of various systems of the body with a person looking on, and do it in a finite time. In reality there is not much more time available for a preoperative assessment of each system in an outpatients or on a ward. At least prepare yourself with a stethoscope. In order to help with making deductions we have provided a number of self tests. These cover some of the common clinical findings and their interpretation.

PHYSICAL EXAMINATION 1 *(Answers on page 77)*

Measuring blood pressure

You are asked to measure the blood pressure and explain the technique.

1. – Blood pressure reading. How will you measure the blood pressure?

2. – Which arm will you measure it in and why?

3. – What is the name of the sounds?

4. – When is systolic pressure taken?

5. – When is diastolic pressure taken?

6. – What are the landmarks of the brachial artery as it enters the antecubital fossa, where the blood pressure is usually taken?

7. – What size of cuff bladder should be used?

8. – What is the effect of using a narrow cuff on an obese patient?

9. – What is the effect of reading the blood pressure in the foot when the patient is supine?

PHYSICAL EXAMINATION 2 (Answers on page 78)

Taking the pulse

1. – What can you tell by examining the radial pulse?

2. – Demonstrate the features of a collapsing pulse.

3. – Name at least three conditions in which the pulse is collapsing.

4. – Demonstrate a modified Allen's test.

5. – What would a positive modified Allen's test be?

6. – What did Allen originally describe the test for?

7. – What is Pulsus alternans?

8. – What is Pulsus paradoxus?

9. – Name three complications of radial arterial catheterisation.

PHYSICAL EXAMINATION 3 *(Answers on page 79)*

You are asked to examine the cardiovascular system.

Start by making sure that the patient is comfortable, undressed to the waist, and lying at about an angle of 45° to the horizontal.

Start with inspection of:

- Hands,
- Pulses,
- Blood pressure,
- Lips or conjunctiva,
- Face,
- Neck,
- Sacrum and ankles,
- Thorax.

Questions

1. – What can be learnt from examining the hands?

2. – What can be learnt from the pulse?

3. – Blood pressure. If the blood pressure is high what will you examine?

4. – What does cyanosis mean?

5. – What may the face show relevant to the CVS?

6. – Look at the neck and the jugular pulse.

   a. How do you differentiate the venous from the carotid pulse?

   b. What are the surface markings of the internal jugular vein?

   c. Describe the normal venous pulse in the neck?

   d. Under what circumstances do you get prominent v wave?

   e. How would you fill the neck veins to demonstrate their presence?

7. – The sacrum and ankles. How does oedema form?

8. – Thorax. Inspect for shape and pulsations. Palpate the precordium.

   What is the normal position of the apex beat?

   What would suggest left or right ventricular enlargement? Some murmurs are palpable as thrills.

9. – Auscultation for heart sounds and murmurs. Try to make a diagnosis before placing the stethoscope on the chest from the inspection and signs already found. What will be the cause of a systolic or a diastolic murmur?

PHYSICAL EXAMINATION 4 *(Answers on page 81)*

Respiratory system

You are asked to demonstrate how to examine the respiratory system.

Questions

1. – What position should the patient be in?

2. – Start by inspection. What are you looking for?

3. – Palpate the trachea position and the apex position. Palpate the chest wall and movement with respiration. What are you feeling for and what may it mean?

4. – Percussion. Think how you will do this with the least fuss. Slow practitioners are those who repeat everything. So get into the habit of placing the hand on to the chest wall and tapping once only in each position. Three taps takes three times as long and if you train your ear three taps will give you no more information than one tap – percuss at the apex and bases right and left. What changes may be detected?

5. – Tactile fremitus or vibration. Place the ulnar side of the hand against the chest wall and ask the patient to say 99. What does an increase mean?

6. – Auscultation. What will this detect?

7. – What simple bed side tests can be performed of lung function?

PHYSICAL EXAMINATION 5 *(Answers on page 83)*

You are asked to examine the cranial nerves

At each stage note how you will make the examination, or do it with a patient or colleague and then check against the relevant answer paragraph.

Examine the cranial nerves.

Questions

How will you test the function of:

1. – First nerve: **Olfactory nerve.**

2. – Second nerve: **Optic nerve.**

3. – Third, fourth and sixth nerves: **Oculomotor, Trochlear and Abducent.**

4. – Fifth cranial nerve: **Trigeminal nerve.**

5. – Seventh nerve: **Facial nerve.**

6. – Eighth nerve: **Auditory and Vestibular nerves.**

7. – Ninth nerve: **Glossopharyngeal nerve.**

8. – Tenth nerve: **Vagus nerve.**

9. – Eleventh nerve: **Accessory nerve.**

10. – Twelfth nerve: **Hypoglossal nerve.**

SELF TEST –
PHYSICAL EXAMINATION 5 *(Answers on page 86)*

Questions

1. – What changes might the eye show in diabetes?

2. – If there is bi-temporal field loss where is the lesion?

3. – What are the features of Horner's syndrome and which nerve(s) is(are) involved?

4. – What does a unilateral ptosis indicate?

5. – An inability to bite properly may be a lesion of which nerve? Which muscle is involved?

6. – Loss of taste to the anterior two thirds of the tongue involves which nerves?

7. – If the conduction is heard best in the right ear when the tuning fork is placed on the forehead but the patient complains of deafness in the right ear what is the problem?

8. – How would you test the functioning of the 9th cranial nerve?

9. – What symptom may indicate a 10th nerve palsy?

10. – Which muscle movements are tested for 11th nerve function?

PHYSICAL EXAMINATION 6   (Answers on page 87)

You are asked to examine the nervous system, apart from the cranial nerves.

Questions

  1. – What tests will you perform of brain stem and cerebellar function?

The peripheral nervous system is divided into:
Efferent – motor function
Afferent – sensory input and
Autonomic nervous system both efferent and afferent

  2. – How will you test motor function?

  3. – How will you test sensory funtion?

SELF TEST –
PHYSICAL EXAMINATION 6 *(Answers on page 89)*

Questions

1. – What position does the arm take up following an upper brachial plexus palsy such as might occur from traction while lying on the operating table?

2. – Which nerve roots are affected if the triceps reflexes are reduced?

3. – What position does the arm assume in a radial nerve palsy, and what is the distribution of loss of sensation?

4. – If there is a sensory level below the clavicles and normal arm function, where is the level of the lesion likely to be?

5. – A sensory level at the umbilicus suggests a lesion at which spinal root?

6. – If the patient is unable to dorsiflex the hallux, which nerve root may be affected?

7. – Numbness on the medial calf can be due to which nerve defect, and which dermatome?

8. – Name 3 causes of Parkinsonism.

9. – The treatment for idiopathic Parkinsonism involves which drugs?

10. – Name three conditions leading to a loss of a knee jerk.

ANSWERS
PHYSICAL EXAMINATION

Measuring blood pressure

1. Practise taking the blood pressure with a mercury sphygmomanometer. You may not have done it for some time. The patient should be positioned so that the arm, cuff and sphygmomanometer are all at the same level as the heart.

2. Measure the pressure in both arms. There may be coarctation of the aorta or an arterio-venous fistula.

3. Korotkoff.

4. First sound.

5. Fifth sound. Except in hyperdynamic states such as seen in pregnancy when the fourth sound is usually taken as the diastolic pressure.

6. Medial to and under the medial border of biceps; medial to the biceps tendon.

7. Cuff bladder length = Twice the width
   Width of the cuff should be the diameter of arm + 20%, or half of the circumference (circumference is about 3 times the diameter (22/7)).

8. It will over read the pressure.

9. The systolic pressure reading will be higher in the foot than if read in the aorta or brachial artery.

Answers – Physical Examination 2

Taking the pulse

1. Rate, rhythm – regular or irregular, volume, the nature of the pulse and the artery wall. You should count the pulse for a full minute if possible or explain that you are doing it for 30 seconds. Feel both radial arteries and if necessary the femoral arteries.

   Atherosclerotic rings may be felt in the arterial wall.

   Small volume pulse pressure: aortic stenosis, low blood pressure or low cardiac output.

2. Collapsing: raise arm above heart to feel the column of blood as if it were transiently banging against the palpating fingers (also called a water hammer pulse).

3. Present with aortic incompetence, hyperdynamic circulation as in thyrotoxicosis, a-v fistulae.

4. Allen's test. Identify radial and ulnar arteries at wrist. Squeeze hand to exsanguinate it. Occlude radial and ulnar arteries – check by seeing pale hand. Release ulnar artery and watch re-perfusion of hand indicating perfusion through a patent ulnar artery and palmar arch vessels in hand.

5. Positive test – no ulnar flow.

6. Allen was originally interested in diagnosing endarteritis obliterans of the digital arteries.

7. Pulsus alternans is alternating strong and weak beats seen in left ventricular failure.

8. The pulse volume normally increases in inspiration due to a reduced intra-thoracic pressure and an increased venous return to the heart; this will give a reduction in heart rate in young fit patients – sinus arrhythmia. The change of heart rate with respiration – beat to beat variation is a sign of competent cardiovascular reflexes and disappears in disease and anaesthesia. Pulsus paradoxus: normally blood pressure changes by 5 to 10mmHg during the respiratory cycle. An increase in this variation in blood pressure occurs in: pericardial effusion and constrictive pericarditis, severe asthma, and gives a pulsus paradoxus.

9. Arterial catheterisation may be complicated by: infection, haemorrhage, arteriovenous fistula, complete occlusion of the artery leading to finger ischaemia and gangrene, embolisation to the finger(s), the injection of incompatible materials.

Answers – Physical Examination 3

Cardiovascular system

1. Finger clubbing can be caused by cyanotic heart disease and infective endocarditis. Other causes include chronic suppurative lung diseases, chronic lower bowel conditions and, cancer of the lung.

   Splinter haemorrhages are seen in trauma, embolisation and subacute endocarditis.

2. Pulse for rate, rhythm, volume nature e.g. collapsing and character of wall.

3. Blood pressure – if hypertensive consider examining the fundus of the eye and other limbs for evidence of coarctation.

4. Cyanosis is a bluish discolouration of the lips, mucous membranes and tongue. This indicates that more than 5 g/100ml of haemoglobin is desaturated.

5. Face. Cyanosis, malar flush.

6. *a.* The venous pulse is seen but not felt; has a double wave, is increased in height by a valsalva manoeuvre and pressure on the liver. The height of the venous pulse wave will alter with posture and goes down with inspiration.

   b. Landmarks for the internal jugular pulse. Deep to sternomastoid. The internal jugular vein runs from the angle of the mandible to a point behind the clavicle about 2 fingers width from the mid-line. The vertical height of filling in the vein above the manubrium–sternal angle may give a measure of the pressure in the right atrium.

   c. The normal venous wave is an "a" wave coinciding with atrial contraction, a "c" wave transmitted from the carotid artery, a "v" wave due to pressure of atrial filling while the tricuspid valve is closed.

   d. Tricuspid incompetence will give a larger "v" wave.

   e. Ask the patient to do a Valsalva manoeuvre to distend the veins, or gently palpate and put pressure on the liver. Ask if the liver is tender first.

7. Oedema occurs when the capillary pressure exceeds the oncotic pressure. A raised right atrial pressure leading to a raised venous pressure will lead to symmetrical peripheral oedema. Venous or lymphatic obstruction will give an asymmetrical oedema. You should know Starling's equation.

8. The apex beat is the furthest point outward and downwards that a cardiac impulse can be felt. It is normally in the mid clavicular line and 5th intercostal space but it will be further out with left ventricular enlargement. Right heart enlargement will cause a lifting of the sternum, or to the left of the sternum detected by the flat of the hand.

9. Auscultation may be used to detect the nature of the first and second sounds as the flow through the valves suddenly changes. Murmurs are due to turbulent flow through a valve. A systolic murmur occurs when the mitral and tricuspid valves should be shut. The commonest cause in the elderly is noise of flow through an arteriosclerotic aorta. It may be back flow through an incompetent mitral or tricuspid valve or a ventricular septal defect or forward flow through a stenosed aortic or pulmonary valve. The murmur of an ASD is the excessive flow of blood through a normal pulmonary valve. Diastolic murmurs occur when the mitral and tricuspid valves are open and the aortic and pulmonary valves closed. Mitral diastolic murmurs are difficult to hear but there are clues that they will be present. The clues are: a history of rheumatic heart disease; the presence of a mitral systolic murmur as stenosis and incompetence often go together; the opening snap after the second sound in diastole and just before the diastolic murmur.

Answers – Physical Examination 4

Respiratory system

1. Sitting comfortably at a 45° incline.

2. Central cyanosis of the mucosa inside the lips and peripheral cyanosis in the fingers. Central cyanosis suggests respiratory failure or a cardiac lesion with a right to left shunt whereas peripheral cyanosis may be a local disorder of the hand. Count the respiratory rate.

   Hands for clubbing. A sign of bronchial cancer, chronic sepsis of the lung such as bronchiectasis. The nicotine staining of the smoker.

   Look for abnormalities of the chest wall. Flattening of part of the chest wall may indicate underlying collapse, fibrosis or past surgery.

   The hyper-expansion of emphysema. Sputum: amount and colour.

3. A shift in the trachea away from the mid line indicates underlying disease. Is it being pushed by tumour or pulled by fibrosis? A shift in the apex beat may mean a shift in the mediastinum.

   Hold your hands against the chest wall with the thumb tips touching over the sternum and watch the movement of breathing. Does one side move more than the other? Repeat at the back of the chest or wait until the patient is sat forward to examine all of the chest from the back, having completed the examination from the front.

4. Percussion leading to resonance suggests hyper-inflation as in emphysema, a pneumothorax – unlikely in the examination. Dullness suggests collapse, consolidation or fibrosis. Very dull suggests fluid in an effusion. Dullness will usually be associated with a shift in the trachea to that side.

5. Tactile fremitus increases in conditions in which the sound is transmitted easily to the periphery of the lung e.g. consolidation.

6. By now you should be expecting to hear something different if it exists. Your examination up to this point should give you a good idea of where the problem is and what your might hear.

   Ask the patient to breathe through the open mouth, otherwise under normal circumstances little will be heard. Normal breathing is silent. You are listening for increased or reduced sounds, and then extra sounds of wheeze or pulmonary secretions, oedema etc. Air sounds will be reduced if the lung is poorly ventilated as in collapse, lung fibrosis, effusion or pneumothorax.

   Bronchial breathing occurs due to the transmission of bronchial or tracheal sounds – that is an equal inspiratory and expiratory sound directly to the periphery through consolidated, collapsed or fibrosed lung. Bronchial breathing is an equal quality of sound during inspiration and expiration.

Added sounds are unlikely in the examination hall as pulmonary oedema and pneumonia patients will not be fit enough to come. So the bronchitic with his cough may have added sounds but check whether they stay after a cough.

7. The healthy patient can blow a flame out at 15 cm with an open mouth and hold their breath for 30 seconds.

    Do you know how to use a simple vitalograph or peak flow meter? Simple peak flow meters are made available to patients with asthma to test their own function.

    Ask the patient to take a maximum breath in and blow out into the device as quickly as possible.

    A normal value should be a PEFR between 400 and 500 l/min for a young adult.

Examination of cranial nerves

1. Test for smell: The response to smell is variable. The test requires specific materials which are unlikely to be available other than in neurological clinics. So this nerve will usually be passed over unless proper samples are available. You might ask about head injury, obvious anosmia or a related change in taste. Otherwise miss this cranial nerve.

2. Test for: *a.* Fundus and visual acuity.

   b. Pupil size and pupillary reflexes.

   c. Visual fields.

   a. Examine the fundus, particularly for changes associated with hypertension and diabetes. Test for blindness by asking the patient to read a few words.

   Test fields of vision for temporal and nasal loss. Temporal loss occurs with pituitary tumours – can you explain how? Variable field losses with multiple sclerosis.

   b. Look at the symmetry of the sizes of the pupils. Exclude Horner's syndrome.

   Reflexes - involving cranial nerves 2 and 3. The pupil should constrict when a light is brought in from the side - indicating a light reflex. The opposite pupil should also constrict indicating a consensual light reflex. Test accommodation by moving an object, such as your finger, in towards the eye from a distance away. The pupil should constrict.

3. Test for: Eye movement - eye and eyelid movement and sympathetic eye innervation.

   Third: Innervates most of the extrinsic eye muscles moving the eye upwards, medially (adduction) and downwards–outwards, also raises the upper lid. The fourth (trochlear) is limited to the superior oblique muscle.

   Test if the patient can look down and inwards. Sixth (abducent) to the lateral rectus muscle.

   Test if the eye moves laterally.

   A ptosis may be unilateral due to:
   • a third nerve palsy with a dilated pupil and eye movement limited to "down and out".
   • a Horner's syndrome with a small pupil.
   • a LMN seventh palsy (see under 7).

   or bilateral due to:
   • myasthenia gravis.
   • myotonia dystrophica

Nystagmus involves several nerve pathways. It consists of a slow movement in one direction and a fast movement back. Its presence may indicate a defect in the cerebellum, brain stem or less commonly the cerebral hemispheres.

Brain death tests involve testing for nystagmus by putting cold water into the ear to test the vestibular nerve. A normal response is a slow movement towards and fast away from the cold stimulus.

4. Test: Sensation of the face.

Three divisions.

Ophthalmic: Forehead including tip of nose – also the cornea.
Maxillary: Cheek from lower eyelid to upper lip including side of nose and palate.

Mandibular: Lower lip and chin.

Test with light touch – cotton wool on cornea and skin, then pin prick to skin.

Also taste to anterior two thirds of tongue from the seventh via the chorda tympani.

Motor fibres to muscles of mastication, particularly masseter. Ask to grin, look for a hollow in the temporal fossa and test by opening the mouth against a resistance. Try biting on a spatula.

5. Test: Motor power to facial muscles:

Ask to grimace by screwing up face, eyes tight closed, raise forehead. Consider the following situations. Distinguish weakness due to an upper motor neurone (UMN) deficit e.g. a CVA; from a lower motor neurone (LMN) weakness of Bell's palsy (a virus infection affecting the facial nerve in the ear). In a LMN lesion the mouth is pulled to the opposite side by a smile and the eye rolls up under the eyelid rather than the eyelid closing tightly on the affected side. The lower neurone lesion affects all of the side of the face including one side of the forehead. In an UMN lesion the forehead muscles contract on both sides, the eyes close and the blinking is preserved due to bilateral upper motor neurone control. Nerve damage due to a parotid lesion or during parotid surgery will give a variable weaknesses. If a ptosis is bilateral consider myasthenia gravis.

6. Test: Hearing by talking into ear or a tuning fork held near to the ear. This also tests the ossicle system in the middle ear. Tuning fork to the mastoid bone tests for a conduction deafness.

Weber's test distinguishes conduction from nerve deafness. A high pitch tuning fork is plucked and then placed against the middle of the forehead. The sound is heard best in the normal ear if nerve deafness, or best in deaf ear if conduction deafness. If heard equally no deafness, or ears equally deaf.

7. Test: Taste to the posterior one third of tongue and by eliciting the gag reflex. Test for difficulty in swallowing.

8. The vagus, or wanderer, innervates the thoracic and abdominal viscera.

Test: The recurrent laryngeal nerve is best tested by observing the movement of the cords at laryngoscopy. Weakness may cause hoarseness or an impaired force to coughing. A nerve weakness may occur at thyroid surgery and with lesions at the apex of the lung.

9. Test: Motor function of sternomastoid and trapezius.

Trapezius. Shrug shoulders. Sternomastoid turn head to one side against resistance.

10. Motor innervation to tongue.

Test: Protrude tongue straight out.

Answers – Self Test 5

1. The eye is affected in a number of ways:
   • Cataracts
   • Retinal haemorrhages and exudates
   • Reduced vision due to macular damage
   • Retinal ischaemia and new vessel formation

2. In the mid line pressing on the centre of the optic chiasma, probably due to a lesion of the pituitary gland, craniopharyngioma, or secondary tumour.

3. Miosis, enophthalmos, ptosis, anhydrosis (plus nasal stuffiness not classically described by Horner). The conjunctival blood vessels may be dilated. All due to a lesion of sympathetic innervation to the head.

4. Lesion of
   • sympathetic innervation, Horner's syndrome,
   • third, or
   • seventh cranial nerve palsy, probably lower motor neurone e.g. Bell's palsy.

5. Fifth cranial nerve and masseter muscle.

6. Seventh cranial nerve via the chorda tympani to the peripheral part of the fifth cranial nerve.

7. A conduction deafness in the right ear.

8. Ask the patient to swallow. Gag reflex elicited if an object is placed towards the back of the mouth or tongue.

9. Hoarseness or a poor force of cough.

10. Trapezius – shrugging of the shoulders. Sternomastoid – rotating the head against a resistance.

Answers – Physical Examination 6

The nervous system

1. Ask the patient to walk a short distance and observe the gait which may indicate: a hemiplegia, stiff and jerky due to spasticity.

   Parkinsonism - small shuffling steps, difficult to start and stop walking, everything appears stiff.

   Test: Stand patient upright with eyes closed. Ask patient to hold hand out level with the face, point the index finger and then bring it to the nose. If the patient fails to bring the finger directly to the nose there is a cerebellar disorder; but exclude a deficit in joint position sense or a motor weakness. Cerebellar disease may be associated with a terminal intention tremor.

   Test: For coordination of upper limb by finger – nose pointing.
   Lower limb by heel – shin slide.
   Rapid, repetitive movement of the hands for disdiadokokinesis.

2. Test motor function

   • Look at the position of the limb for an obvious palsy; then look at the muscles for wasting and fasciculations.

   • Palpate the muscle tone which can be flaccid with a lower motor neurone lesion. Increased tone can be either clasp knife: that is stiff to start with and then gives way in cerebral lesions like a CVA, or cogwheel: that is stiff throughout as in Parkinsonism with a pill rolling tremor which stops when doing something.

   • Reflexes

   Test the nerve arc from stretch receptors to spinal cord and back to muscle.
   Upper limb: Biceps (C5, 6), Triceps (C7, 8), Brachio radialis (C5, 6).
   Lower limb: Knee (L4) and Ankle (S1). Dorsiflexion of the hallux depends on L5.

   Know the dermatomes of each reflex tested. An absent ankle reflex may not be significant in the elderly.

   Plantar reflex. The stimulus should be applied along the lateral border of the foot. In the presence of an upper motor neurone lesion, such as in the pyramidal tracts, the big toe extends. Stimulating the sole of the foot will produce a withdrawal reflex.

3. Tests of sensory function.

   • Light touch and vibration pass in the dorsal columns on the same side of the spinal cord, only crossing to the other side in the medulla.

   • Pain with temperature pass to the contralateral anterior lateral spino-thalamic tracts.

Test with cotton wool for light touch and a tuning fork on boney promontories for vibration sense. Test for pain and cold with a pin and an alcohol wipe. Test on the trunk for a sensory level with a cold alcohol wipe.

Typically in syringomyelia pain is lost on one side and light touch on the other.

Test both pain and light touch for loss of dermatome innervation and for specific nerve distribution. For instance: an ulnar nerve palsy will give loss of sensation to the palm and dorsum of the hand affecting the little finger and the ulnar half of the ring finger. In a C8 dermatome lesion the sensory loss will extend up the forearm to the antecubital fossa on the ulnar side.

Answers – Self Test 6

1. Upper trunk paralysis C5 affects the muscles: deltoid, biceps, brachioradialis and brachialis. The arm hangs down by the side, medially rotated, forearm extended and pronated. Shoulder abduction and elbow flexion is lost. This is Erb's palsy or waiters tip position.

   A lower trunk C8 T1 paralysis affects the small muscles of the hand and flexion of the wrist and fingers is lost. The unchecked extension gives a claw hand or Klumpke's palsy.

2. C 7 and 8.

3. Radial nerve lesion.
   Motor loss leads to lack of hand extension and so a dropped wrist.
   Sensory loss on the dorsum of the hand on the radial side.

   Median nerve lesion.
   Motor loss produces an ape like hand with lack of thenar muscle action and flexion of the hand may be weak.
   Sensory loss of palmar surface of hand and fingers except for the little finger and part of the ring finger.

   Ulnar nerve lesion.
   Motor loss is an inability to stretch out the fingers and hypothenar wasting. The hand appears clawed.
   Sensory loss over the ulnar side of the hand on palmar and dorsal surfaces.

4. T2.

5. T10.

6. L5.

7. The skin over the medial calf is supplied by the saphenous nerve, a branch of the femoral nerve. Dermatome L4.

8. Idiopathic loss of dopamine neurotransmitter in the substantia nigra, postencephalitic, drug induced e.g. phenothiazines – particularly piperazines, butyrophenones.

9. Drugs: Dopaminergic e.g. levodopa with dopa-decarboxylase, monoamine-oxidase B inhibitors selegiline. Antimuscarinic orphenadrine and benzhexol. Muscle relaxant and anti tremor drugs e.g. diazepam.

10. Damage to the nerve root of L4; multiple sclerosis; causes of myopathies e.g. inflammation, alcohol, hypokalaemia; causes of peripheral neuropathies, diabetes, malignancy, Guillain-Barré syndrome, toxicity: regional anaesthesia and during recovery from general anaesthesia.

COMMUNICATION   **5**

INTRODUCTION

Communication requires various skills including:

- Knowledge.
- The ability to organise your thoughts quickly into a logical order.
- Tact and time to explain a difficult point.

The ability to impart information also requires:

- An awareness about how we communicate.
- What makes for good communication.

A distinction can be drawn between verbal communication and body language. In every day life we use our bodies to convey over half (some estimate up to 80%) of the message that we wish to give to other people. The way in which we use our eyes to make eye contact or to avoid the other person; the way that we sit; the way that we move our hands and body, all convey meaning to the person watching us.

There are various forms of communication such as social chat; a lecture imparting information; an interview for advice or for a job; a vicar in church or a judge in a court of law imparting doctrine, a judgement or condemnation; and a salesman trying to sell a product. Each of these entail a different relationship between the interviewer and the interviewee, the lecturer and the lectured, the salesman and the client.

In the medical interview there is a relationship to be established. Appearance is communicating something about yourself. Punctuality indicates something about commitment as does paying attention or fidgeting. A proper introduction sets the scene. First impressions count for a great deal. In order to establish a rapport with the patient you should appear clean and tidy and in keeping with their expectation of what a professional person should look like. Dressing up may make the patient feel that you are unapproachable or too confident. If a doctor is dirty or shabby, however competent and caring they are underneath, a false impression may be made which prejudices further rapport. When working with children different dress may be appropriate to reduce anxiety. In the examination, as in real life, it is best to wear what you feel most comfortable in and is practical. Bear in mind that you are going to be asked to demonstrate resuscitation skills on a manikin and other skills which may involve you moving quickly around.

Communication is not one skill. In the doctor – patient relationship there are a number of situations which require different communication skills. History taking is the skill of obtaining as much information as possible, relevant to the situation and from that information formulating a differential diagnosis about the condition of the patient.

The anaesthetic communication station can test a number of skills related to dealing with information.

The station may involve:

- Identifying the problem(s) that is (are) giving cause for concern.
- Explaining, in an understandable way, a situation, worry or plan of management.
- Giving information about a clinical situation, suitable for informed consent.
- Dealing with a difficult clinical dilemma.

There is not time during a 5 minute station to offer comfort, support, empathy and other counselling skills. The original meaning of counselling is the process of helping the patient understand their situation better and, with them, to formulate a plan of action. Counselling is used here to mean information skills; informing the patient what will happen, what is available, or what needs to be done, based on the available factual information.

In practice (but in the OSCE there may not be time), in discussing more difficult issues "the my child test" may be helpful. This is to consider that what you are saying or doing is going to be said or done to your child (mother, wife, father, husband etc). If you are happy for it to be said to your child then it is probably good practice; if you would not do it that way to your child, then there is something odd about it.

In the examples that follow you are expected to:

- Find out what the person is concerned about.
- Determine why they are concerned and then give an explanation that will answer their worries.
- Explain a procedure.
- Obtain consent.
- Deal with a difficult clinical situation.

Each question is followed by an opportunity to think of possible avenues before proceeding to the next step. Think of what you would say and the way that you might say it?

To have thought about it is to be prepared.

Try to get a friend to act the part by reading the scenario note at the beginning of the answer to each case and the whole explanatory text with answers. Allow yourself only five minutes and then compare how much you were able to cover of the relevant information.

CASE 1

(Answers on page 101)

You are to see the wife of a patient. Her husband was admitted 6 hours ago following a massive cerebral haemorrhage confirmed by brain scan and his lungs are being ventilated.

Use the 90 seconds in the waiting period to mentally rehearse some of the issues involved.

Introduce yourself.

In real life it is important to check that you are speaking to the right person, before discussing confidential information.

Establish the background. You may be in a hurry but allow time to find out about the situation from the patient's point of view.

– *"Tell me what you know of what has happened."* or

– *"What have you been told so far?"*

The lady says that she knows that ther husband has no hope of recovery.

Questions

1. – Write down the first point(s) that you think is(are) relevant and how you will deal with it(them).

2. – What are the main issues that you will cover?

The lady wants assurance that he is dead.

3. – What will you say?

She has accepted your explanation. Move to the next issue.

4. – What has to be discussed after brain death tests?

In these circumstances it may be necessary to consult the coroner.

5. – What will you say about the coroner?

Finish by offering sympathy and express sadness at what has happened.

CASE 2

(Answers on page 102)

You are to see a mother who is anxious about her son. The son is to have an anaesthetic for insertions of grommets.

Remember that this as an exercise in four parts.

- Find out what has to be explained. In this case what is the cause of the anxiety.
- Find out why it is a problem and what is already known or understood.
- Give a clear explanation to relieve the anxiety.
- Check that there are no other problems and that the explanation has been accepted. Do not go into the situation with any preconceived ideas. This means do not explain something that the patient is not concerned about and miss their problem in the process.

Take the 90 seconds between stations to consider what issues might be causes for anxiety.

Questions

1. – List the possible reasons for anxiety.

   Introduction –You should say who you are, ask their name.

   Rapport and a little background information. Establish a rapport by checking the name and age of the child. Then go straight to the point. *"Tell me about your anxiety,"* or *"What are you most concerned about?"*.

   Ask open ended questions. That is questions that cannot easily be answered by a Yes or No reply. Allow the person to tell you, preferably without interruption, about their problem.

The mother is concerned because her nephew did not recover from an operation six years ago.

2. – At this point formulate a list of possible explanations.

   You may need to clarify whether he died or was recovery delayed?

   "Tell me more about your nephew." "What do you mean by saying he did not recover?" The nephew had a tonsillectomy but did not breathe properly after surgery. In recovery he was ventilated for 3 hours before waking up. You may have to clarify with the mother that it was due to the muscle relaxant.

You are now expected to explain suxamethonium apnoea to this mother.

3. – What points would you cover?

94

The mother may have a second concern about leaving her son in the operating theatre. This gives you a lead to explain the preparation for theatre.

4. – What points will you cover?

Finally, before leaving, reassure her that she is welcome to come to the theatre and check that she understands what will happen. Check that there are no other concerns.

CASE 3

(Answers on page 104)

You are asked to discuss consent for anaesthesia with a Jehovah's witness who needs a hysterectomy.

Do not forget to start by introducing yourself. Then quickly get to the main problem as indicated by the instruction card. Problem of operating on a Jehovah's witness.

Clarify the main problem. "*Tell me exactly how your belief affects surgery.*"

Questions

1. – What issue(s) is(are) likely to be a problem?

2. – What options will you consider once you have established the patient's view?

3. – What are the other issues that need clarifying pre-operatively from the introduction?

CASE 4

(Answers on page 105)

The patient is a Greek or a West Indian who is due to have an inguinal hernia repaired. Introduce yourself and then ask about any general health problems. The patient says that he has no knowledge of any blood diseases in his family, he is well but has lost a little weight. He is a policeman. Explain the need for a sickle test. He is not keen on needles.

Questions

1. – What is(are) the relevant issue(s) that may need to be discussed?

Write down what you might expect to talk about.

2. – What will you pursue now?

He still does not want a blood test.

3. – Why would he not want a blood test?

The patient gives a history of weight loss.

4. – What will you ask about?

The patient is Sickledex positive.

5. – How will you proceed?

CASE 5

(Answers on page 106)

You are told that the patient is having a hysterectomy and is concerned about pain relief.

Questions

1. – What are the issues?

   Introduce yourself and immediately allow the patient to tell you about their problem. *"What is their anxiety?"* *"Is there a particular reason for being anxious?"*

2. – *"What would you like to know about pain relief?"* What strategy will you follow for postoperative pain relief?

3. – What will you explain about PCA?

4. – Do intramuscular injections have a place?

5. – What else will you give with the PCA?

6. – What else might be given?

   Finally you may have to help the patient choose what to have.

   "What do you advise doctor?"

7. – Your choice is...

CASE 6

(Answers on page 108)

The patient is concerned about a proposed operation for varicose veins.

Introduction – always introduce yourself by name.

This is a specific station about communication therefore ask the patient what their concern is. Take your lead from the introductory note "*is concerned*".

Questions

   1. – What might the patient be concerned about?

In this case the patient had a tonsillectomy as a child and remembers being awake while things were being done inside the mouth.

It is not unusual for patients to mention awareness years later when they come for a second operation.

They may not have mentioned it at the time.

   2. – What will your response include?

   3. – What conditions will you try to exclude as possible reasons for what has happened?

The patient wants reassurance about this anaesthetic. They say that their mother was told that there was a fault in the apparatus last time.

   4. – What will you say?

Before finishing always check if there are any other concerns.

In an examination it is possible to ask the actor to add another concern.

This patient says they are still frightened of dying during the anaesthetic.

   5. – What will you say?

CASE 7

(Answers on page 110)

You are asked to see a pregnant lady seeking advice about pain relief.

Start with an introduction and ask what advice is required. The lady says she is anxious about having pain in labour.

Questions

1. – What do you want to know?

Patient says that she is concerned about having a lot of pain.
She would like an epidural.

2. – How will you respond?

She wishes to know more about an epidural for labour.

3. – What will you say?

The patient decides that she wants to know about the other methods.

4. – Which methods will you mention?

The patient may be undecided and ask which technique you recommend.

5. – What will you say?

ANSWERS
COMMMUNICATION

Answers – CASE 1

Relative's scenario: Play the part of a person whose spouse has been admitted following a cerebral haemorrhage and whose life is only supported by a ventilator. You want to know if s/he is dead.

1. What does the person already know. What do they want explained.

2. A. Brain death tests and turning off the ventilator. The involvement of the relative in the decision to turn off a ventilator is difficult. The turning off of a ventilator is a medical decision. The relative does not have medical knowledge, but they do have feelings, which in these circumstances are confused. In grief the relative will not necessarily be able to make rational decisions. For one partner to die is a threat to the very existence of the remaining partner who is not going to want to be put into the situation of turning off their own life. The reasons for turning off have to be explained to the relative.

   B. Potential donor – card carrier

   C. Refer the case to the coroner.

3. Explain the procedures for brain death tests, in the presence of a known diagnosis. Stop all drugs. Normal body chemistry and temperature. A series of tests of brain function. All tests done by two doctors. No pupil movement, no eye movement, no spontaneous breathing, no response to pain. If no response present then all tests repeated. Explain peripheral movements due to spinal reflexes.

4. Deal with the possibility of the patient being a donor. Is s/he a potential donor? Was s/he in good health? The question of testing for HIV and hepatitis should be mentioned. Did s/he carry a donor card or express any wish? Indicate the organs that might be used: kidney, heart, lungs, liver, pancreas, corneas. Perhaps introduce the idea that someone else may be helped out of their tragedy.

5. Explain the role of the coroner in establishing cause of death, when death is sudden or suspicious. Some coroners will want to be informed when donation is involved or if there has been an industrial disease. Explain that the coroner may want to talk to them. Reassure them that this is not a court of law, s/he is not looking for blame.

Answers – CASE 2

Parent scenario: You are a parent of a child who is to have an operation. You are worried about his anaesthetic as your nephew had a tonsillectomy and needed ventilation for some 3 hours postoperatively. You know that it was something to do with a muscle relaxant called suxamethonium. A second issue is that you want to know what will happen on the day of surgery.

1. Previous operations with complications; congenital or acquired conditions; family illness or death; present condition.

2. Inherited conditions that might present in childhood (not many children have acquired diseases in early life). Suxamethonium apnoea, porphyria, malignant hyperpyrexia and congenital conditions of CVS, CNS, and cystic fibrosis. Trauma associated with an accident. Anaphylactic conditions are rare in children. A relative overdose of local anaesthetic or opiate are possibilities. Establish exactly what happened. If it was a congenital condition is there a blood relationship to this child?

3. Explain the nature of suxamethonium, commonly used to secure the airway. Defective gene inherited from mother and father which then leads to a failure to produce the normal enzyme needed to destroy this drug quickly. There is a slower route for elimination of the drug, hence the 3 hour delay in recovery. Treatment: maintain respiratory support and sleep while recovery occurs. If there is concern about this child he and other members of the family need testing for the presence of pseudocholinesterase. Give the incidence of the atypical gene 3:10,000 and explain that it runs in families but may not affect her child. If necessary you will not give suxamethonium or mivacurium.

   Other possible scenarios but associated with a longer recovery and residual effects would be: The relative might have presented with abdominal pain, had an appendicectomy which was normal, but the abdominal pain was a presentation of porphyria or diabetes. If porphyria: establish a blood relationship and whether other family members are affected. Porphyria can be difficult to diagnose unless the person is having an attack. There are a limited number of drugs that are relatively safe to give. These include: muscle relaxants, opiates, nitrous oxide, volatile agents, local anaesthetics and benzodiazepines.

   Malignant hyperpyrexia is rare, even in children, 1:14000. Any relative of a MH patient can be investigated at a specialist centre by exposing a muscle biopsy to caffeine or halothane.

   Anaphylaxis. If a person is likely to be allergic to a drug, skin tests can be used to try to define which drugs should be avoided.

4. You will see her child: general health and development, look for loose teeth, assess airway and a possible venous access. EMLA cream, possible oral premedication. Fluids to drink up to 2 hours before the operation. Come to theatre in any clothes, with toy, with one parent to the anaesthetic room. Attach monitors, either a venous or inhalation induction whichever seems appropriate depending on the ease of venous access and airway. Once asleep the parent will leave with a nurse. Explain postoperative pain relief, opiates, NSAI, suppositories and local anaesthesia if relevant and return to drinking. Indicate that the mother can come to the recovery room.

Answers – CASE 3

Patient scenario: Play the part of a Jehovah's witness requiring a hysterectomy for menorrhagia.

1. A Jehovah's witness is unlikely to agree to a blood transfusion. You will need to clarify whether the objection is to:

   a. donor blood,

   b. pre donated blood,

   c. autologous blood such as with bypass surgery.

   You might say:

   – *"Am I correct in assuming that you would rather die than have a blood transfusion?"*

   – *"Would you be happy with me taking some of your own blood out at the beginning of the operation and returning it later if needed. It will be in contact with you all the time."* The contact may be acceptable to some.

   – *"Which fluids are you happy to receive?"* This will probably be limited to crystalloid and colloid derived from non blood sources such as dextran and starch products. Indicate that you will seek senior help.

2. There are a number of options.

   a. Transfer to doctor/hospital specialising in these cases. Indicate that you will consult with other colleagues and look for senior surgical involvement.

   b. Explain ways to minimise blood loss: epidural and spinal anaesthesia, hypotensive techniques with direct arterial pressure monitoring.

   c. Obtain written consent and write in the patient's notes any details such as refusing to have blood. Get the patient to sign the details of the consent in the notes. Make sure the relatives know what is happening.

3. The reason for the hysterectomy. Is it life saving e.g. for cancer or menorrhagia? Is the patient anaemic? Would they benefit from treatment e.g. iron sulphate?

Answers – CASE 4

Patient scenario: Play the part of a Greek, Indian or African who might have sickle or thalassaemia disease but has also lost some weight. You work as a policeman. You are frightened of doctors and needles.

1. Mediterranean patients and those from Africa, or of African descent, have the possibility of having sickle cell disease or thalassaemia. 25% of Africans carry the sickle call gene. Sickle disease is also prevalent in certain parts of India and the Far East.

2. Four issues:
   a. The weight loss, in the absence of symptoms. Has he got a chronic infection – hepatitis, tuberculosis; a cancer; metabolic disorder such as diabetes?
   b. Why is he frightened of needles? You might offer a small needle and EMLA cream.
   c. The inguinal hernia can be associated with an intra-abdominal tumour.
   d. Always ask about occupation. How might it be relevant?

3. He may fear a test revealing a disease which would exclude him from his job such as hepatitis, epilepsy, AIDS, illegal drugs – steroids for sports or recreational drugs, high alcohol intake.

   How will you deal with this?

   Indicate that the test is only for sickle cell disease. Is he frightened of being tested for anything else? It might be important to know if he has other diseases such as AIDS or hepatitis. Reassure him that nothing else is tested without his consent, if it is not relevant to the present condition.

4. How much weight have you lost and over how many weeks? Is it deliberate: Are you on a diet? Ask about any other symptoms such as malaise, tiredness, pyrexia or lumps. Think of infection, cancer or diabetes.

5. The sickledex test does not differentiate trait from disease. The blood should be tested by electrophoreses and if the disease is present consider a local anaesthetic technique – epidural or spinal. Avoid tourniquets. Check whether there is a contraindication such as a clotting problem, back infection and obtain consent. Then be prepared to explain the details of an epidural: iv access and fluids with BP monitoring, position, risk 1:100 of post spinal tap headache. Leg weakness and numbness, retention of urine.

Answers – CASE 5

Patient scenario: Play the part of a patient who is to have abdominal surgery and is anxious to have good pain relief.

1. This is a scenario about postoperative pain relief. The patient may have experienced pain in previous operations. Do not wander off into other areas without dealing with this worry first.

2. This requires a logical method of explanation. *"There are many different methods of relieving pain, do you want to know about all of them?"*

   Balanced analgesia should include: Opiates as PCA or IM, Local anaesthetics, NSAIDs, Entonox, Transcutaneous nerve stimulation (TENS).

3. What will you say about PCA?

   Explain how it works. You press a button and the device gives you a small dose. You can titrate the total dose against your pain and any side effects. Side effects: some sedation, nausea and vomiting – you will have an antiemetic. Because the peaks in the doses are less the nausea and itch (if it occurs) should be less severe.

   There is a short lock out of up to 10 minutes before taking another dose, to give the previous dose time to work. So you cannot give yourself too much, nor can you become addicted. Only you should press the button.

4. Intramuscular injections are still used. *"There may be nausea which can usually be treated with an antiemetic. If you require a limited number of doses this is a method to consider. If you prefer the nurse to give you pain relief, then you can call the nurse or they will come and ask you if you have any pain and give you an appropriate dose of morphine when you ask. Do not keep quiet and suffer in silence, make sure you ask the nurse for a dose when you need it, you will not become addicted."*

   Intramuscular drugs are best given by the nurse asking the patient every hour whether or not they have pain. Reassure the patient that nausea will be dealt with and addiction is not a problem.

5. Give an anti-inflammatory drug. This can be given as a wafer onto the tongue, as a suppository, or by injection. There are a number of conditions when non steroidal anti-inflammatory drugs may not be advisable and there is a need to check that the patient does not have: peptic ulcers, renal impairment, asthma with nasal polyps, liver disease, or a clotting problem. *"I will give you a dose of non steroidal before you wake up."* *"These drugs are good as the sole analgesic after any severe pain is easing and when you can take oral medication."*

   Obtain informed consent before using a suppository and warn about anal discharge. Record your advice in the patient's notes.

6. Local anaesthetics, particularly if the patient has a problem with opiates or NSAIDs.

    There are a number of different local anaesthetic techniques that can be used, either single dose, top ups or continuous infusions to give longer relief.

    Explain that: *"Normally a dose of local anaesthetic is placed into and around the wound before you wake up. This will make it numb for a few hours. Consider an epidural. There are more potential problems than with the other techniques and it requires more intensive nursing postoperatively."*

    "An epidural can be continued into the postoperative period but the legs may be numb and weak and the bladder may not function normally. There is a risk of a headache due to a dural tap and low CSF pressure. The blood pressure can go down so you need a drip; we have to be careful to observe your breathing closely after the operation and you may get an itch if an opiate is mixed with the local anaesthetic."

    If you are thinking of an epidural do not forget to warn the patient of headache incidence 1:100, bladder weakness and retention of urine, and if using opiates – respiratory problems and itch.

7. Find out which one the patient might prefer.

    If they do not know, offer your best method. *"I would recommend a balanced method: an anti-inflammatory and opiate drug while you are asleep and local anaesthetic into the wound before you wake up. A PCA device with an antiemetic once you are awake enough to press the button."*

    The test is to cover all the information in an organised way.

Answers – CASE 6

Patient scenario: Play the part of patient who was aware during a childhood tonsillectomy and is to have a varicose vein operation. You are also frightened of dying during a general anaesthetic.

1. Concern might be about awareness, fear of not waking up or death, nausea and vomiting, pain. Whatever the concern is, ask why? Has something affected them, a relative or friend or have they read an article.

2.   *a.* Show some sympathy.

     b. Find out when the awareness happened. Patients may remember the intubation if there is a delay and the effect of induction agents is passing off. Think – was this a difficult intubation?

     c. The patient may be aware during the operation for various reasons. Emergency situations such as severe hypotension may mean 100% oxygen was given. There may have been a faulty anaesthetic machine, ventilator or a vaporiser became empty. The later implies a lack of monitoring.

     d. It may have happened in recovery if there was a problem with the airway postoperatively. Ascertain whether the patient could move or were they paralysed?

     e. Were they in pain or did they hear a conversation?

   Impress on everyone that you are taking the situation seriously, getting all the facts. Have they had any subsequent operations with or without problems?

3. Try to exclude an anaphylaxis reaction – do you have an 'alert' disc for an allergy?, difficult intubation with delay. If the awareness was in recovery was the anaesthetic prolonged and why? Exclude a suxamethonium apnoea ventilated without sedation. Indicate that you will send for the notes of his operation.

4. How will you proceed for this operation?

     a. Would you consider a local anaesthetic for this operation? Before committing yourself to a local anaesthetic make sure that there are no contraindications: patient willing, anatomy not abnormal, no coagulation problems, no sepsis.

     b. an amnesic premedication before this operation.

     c. if a GA: Reassure that you will stay with patient all the time. Full monitoring including anaesthetic agent concentration. Avoid paralysis or use minimum paralysis so that patient can indicate awareness.

5. Determine the cause for concern. Is there a reason for the fear? Their mother died during an anaesthetic. If possible find the medical notes. What were the circumstances? Is there a link? You are seeking a precise explanation.

It may be necessary to exclude an inherited or an allergic condition.

Has anyone else in your family died or been abnormally ill following an anaesthetic.?

Have you excluded suxamethonium apnoea, anaphylaxis, or rare conditions such as: porphyria, malignant hyperpyrexia, or cardiomyopathy?

Answers – CASE 7

Patient scenario: Play the part of a pregnant lady who is concerned about pain relief in labour. You want an epidural but have had attacks of abdominal pain, suggesting an abruption.

1. Why is she anxious? Has she had a previous painful labour, or has a relative or friend had pain? What does she know about pain relief and has she got an opinion as to what she wants?

2. Do not fall into the trap of offering an epidural without checking the obstetric history.

   Ask about:
   - Number of weeks pregnant.
   - History of bleeding.
   - Previous caesarean section.
   - Back operations.
   - Pain or deformity.
   - Neurological condition especially multiple sclerosis.
   - Back infection.
   - Blood coagulation problem.

3. Explain what an epidural involves: an intravenous infusion in case of fall in blood pressure, lie on side or sit up, injection and catheter to back. Problems with hypotension, loss of bladder control, leg weakness, and loss of sensation below waist. Often a shortened first stage but prolonged second stage. Headache if dural puncture 1:100. It may not be possible if the anatomy is difficult, bleeding indicates abruption or placenta praevia, or pain indicating abruption.

4. You should be prepared to discuss a range of analgesic techniques including: TENS, relaxation, Entonox, intramuscular and intravenous analgesia and PCA when epidural analgesia is not possible.

   Obstetric analgesia is about pain relief in labour not just an epidural service.

5. You may have to give advantages and disadvantages or an opinion.

   Think of issues such as: would an epidural be an advantage to the mother or baby – does she have diabetes, heart condition, pre eclampsia, or is there a multiple pregnancy, breech or premature baby?

   What are the person's expectations about severity of pain. Local anaesthetics are the only technique to completely remove pain but some mothers feel disappointed that they have not had real labour, others may not want the side effects. The options can be left open to choice when the labour starts, and changed if needed.

RESUSCITATION 6

RESUSCITATION 1 (Answers on page 117)

Basic life support

You are asked to demonstrate basic life support on an adult or paediatric manikin with an examiner present.

You would be expected to demonstrate:
1. – Safe approach

2. – Calling for help

3. – Correct sequence of assessment of ABC

4. – Institution of CPR

5. – Airway clearing manoeuvres

6. – Effective mouth to mouth ventilation

7. – Correct position of hands for cardiac massage

8. – Effective compressions at appropriate rate

9. – Correct compression to ventilation ratio.

You may then be asked to complete one of a number of advanced life support protocols relevant to a particular ECG.

RESUSCITATION 2

(Answers on page 118)

Complete the protocol for an adult with ventricular fibrillation.

1. _____

2. _____

3. _____

4. _____

5. _____ + _____ **(if not already)**

6. _____

7. _____

8. _____

9. _____

10. _____

After 3 loops consider. 11. _____

12. _____

NB   Give charges for each defibrillation.
      Give drug dosages.

RESUSCITATION 3

(Answers on page 119)

Complete the protocol for an adult with asystole.

1. _____

2. _____ ?   **if Yes** →

if No ↓

3. _____

4. _____

5. _____

6. _____ + _____ **(if not already)** ←

7. _____

8. _____

9. _____

10. _____ ? **if No** →

if Yes ↓

11. _____

After 3 cycles consider   **12.** _____

RESUSCITATION 4

(Answers on page 120)

Complete the protocol for an adult with electromechanical dissociation.

Consider and treat

1. _____

2. _____

3. _____

4. _____

5. _____

6. _____

7. _____

Then:

8. _____ + _____ (if not already)

9. _____

10. _____

RESUSCITATION 5

(Answers on page 121)

Complete the protocol for a child with ventricular fibrillation.

1.   _____

2.   _____

3.   _____

4.   _____

5.   _____   +   _____   (if not already)

6.   _____

7.   _____

8.   _____

9.   _____

10. _____

11. _____

Consider causes of ventricular fibrillation:

12. _____

13. _____

14. _____

After 3 loops consider:

15. _____

16. _____

RESUSCITATION 6

(Answers on page 122)

Complete the protocol for a child with asystole.

1. _____ + _____

2. _____

3. _____

4. _____

5. _____

Consider:

6. _____

7. _____

ANSWERS
RESUSCITATION

Source: Guidelines for basic life support. BMJ 12th June 1993 pages 1587-1589.
    Read this for a detailed description.

In short, the guidelines are:

1. Approach with caution.
2. Assess responsiveness.
3. Shout for help.
4. Check ABC.–   Open the airway and clear obvious obstructions.
                      Look listen and feel for breathing 5 seconds.
                      Feel for carotid pulse 5 seconds.
5. If breathing and pulse present put in recovery position.
6. If pulse present but no breathing ventilate for 10 breaths then go for help before continuing.
7. If pulse and breathing absent go for help first then start CPR.

    CPR for the adult.

    The correct position for chest compression is over the lower third of the serum in the mid-line. Use two hands and depress 4-5 centimetres at a rate of 80 per minute. The ratio of compressions to ventilations should be 15:2 for a single person or 5:1 if there are two. With each breath aim to give 800-1200 ml, taking one second for each inspiration and allowing two seconds for expiration.

    CPR for child.

    For a child follow steps 1,2 and 3 above. In 4 do not use finger sweep to clear secretions as more damage may occur. If no breathing give 5 breaths then feel for pulse. This is easier to feel in the brachial artery in infants. If no pulse over 1 year or under 60 bpm in infant up to 1 year give CPR at a heart rate of 100 bpm and ratio of 5:1.

    For heart massage in infants use 2 fingers, 1 finger breadth below the inter-nipple line, and depress 2 cm. In the older child use the heel of the hand 2 cm above the xiphoid, and depress 3 cm. After 20 cycles call for emergency services. To ventilate an infant under one year old, the adult mouth surrounds the infant's mouth and nose. Over one year old cover the child's mouth with the adult mouth and pinch the nose. Sufficient volume is forced in to see the chest rise. The adult should take a normal breath each time to maintain a high oxygen content in the exhaled or dead space air.

Answer – RESUSCITATION 2

Source: Adult advanced cardiac life support. BMJ 12th June 1993 pages 1589-1593.

1. Precordial thump

2. DC shock 200 J

3. DC shock 200 J

4. DC shock 360 J

5. Intubate   +   IV access if not already in place.

6. 1 mg adrenaline

7. 10 x 5:1 CPR sequences

8. DC shock 360 J

9. DC shock 360 J

10. DC shock 360 J

After 3 loops consider.   11.   Alkalising agents

                           12.   Anti arrhythmics.

1. Precordial thump if
a) witnessed collapse or b) unable to exclude ventricular fibrillation.

2. VF excluded ?　　**if Yes** →

if No ↓

3. DC shock 200J

4. DC shock 200J

5. DC shock 360J

6. Intubate　　+　　IV access if not already in place

7. Adrenaline 1mg

8. 10 x 5:1 CPR sequences

9. Atropine 3mg (once only)

10. Electrical activity present　?　**if No** →

if Yes ↓

11. Pace

After 3 cycles consider　　**12.** Adrenaline 5 mg

Answers – RESUSCITATION 4

Consider and treat

1. Hypovolaemia

2. Hypothermia

3. Tension pneumothorax

4. Cardiac tamponade

5. Drug overdose

6. Electrolyte imbalance

7. Pulmonary embolus

Then:

8. Intubate   +   IV access   (if not already) ⬅

9. 1 g adrenaline

10. CPR sequences 5:1 x 10 ➡

Answers – RESUSCITATION 5

1. Precordial thump

2. DC shock 2J/kg

3. DC shock 2J/kg

4. DC shock 4J/kg

5. Intubate
   Ventilate 100% oxygen IV   +   Intraosseous access   (if not already)

6. Adrenaline 10 µg/kg

7. CPR for 1 minute

8. DC shock 4J/kg

9. DC shock 4J/kg

10. DC shock 4J/kg

11. Adrenaline 100 µg/kg

Consider causes of ventricular fibrillation:

12. Electrolyte imbalance

13. Drugs

14. Hypothermia

After 3 loops consider:

15. Alkalising agents

16. Anti arrhythmics

Answers – RESUSCITATION 6

1. Intubate   +   ventilate 100% oxygen

2. Intravenous / intraosseous access

3. Adrenaline 10 μg/kg

4. CPR 3 minutes

5. Adrenaline 100 μg/kg

Consider:

6. Fluids

7. Ankalising agents

No precordial thump is recommended in children because vf is rare.

APPARATUS

7

APPARATUS 1

(Answers on page 143)

Tracheal tube

Questions

1. – A nasal tube has the same curvature as an oral tube.   True   False

2. – A nasal tube can be identified by having a longer pilot tube.   True   False

3. – Murphy's eye is to prevent one lung anaesthesia.   True   False

4. – A reinforced tube will not kink.   True   False

5. – The low pressure cuff is designed to only produce a complete seal during inspiration in positive pressure ventilation   True   False

6. – A tube of larger internal diameter will have a greater resistance to spontaneous breathing than a narrow tube.   True   False

7. – Resistance to flow in a tube is inversely related to viscosity.   True   False

8. – The correct length for a tracheal tube is related to the distance from the tragus to the side of the mouth.   True   False

9. – The diameter of the tube in children is given by 4mm or 4.5mm + 1/4 age   True   False

10. – A red rubber tube is more likely than a PVC tube to be ignited by a laser beam.   True   False

APPARATUS 2

(Answers on page 144)

One lung anaesthesia

Write out a sequence for inserting the double lumen tube and inflating the cuffs.

Then check that one lung can be inflated independently of the other.

Use the labels on the diagram opposite to identify each step.

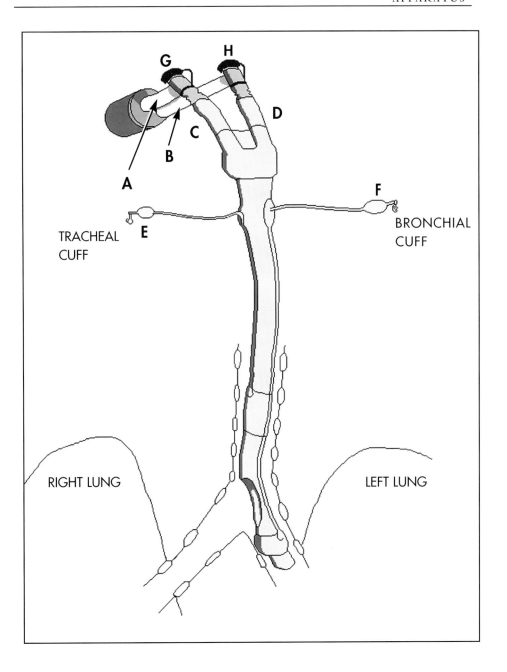

G H

D

A B C

TRACHEAL
CUFF E

F

BRONCHIAL
CUFF

RIGHT LUNG LEFT LUNG

APPARATUS 3

(Answers on page 145)

Nuffield ventilator

A Bain circuit has been connected to a Nuffield ventilator for IPPV as shown. opposite. A fresh gas flow of 6 l/min is set.

Questions

1. – The flow of anaesthetic gas that the patient receives from the anaesthetic machine will not be diluted by oxygen, or other driving gas, if the volume of the connecting tubing from the ventilator up to the patient is 500ml.   True   False

2. – The rate of ventilation will be 12 breaths per minute.   True   False

3. – The I:E ratio is set at 1:2.   True   False

4. – The tidal volume will be 1000ml (1 litre).   True   False

5. – The expired gas will be void to a scavenger at point A.   True   False

6. – The connections at point C are 22mm in diameter.   True   False

7. – A fresh gas flow of 70ml/kg/min and IPPV with the parameters set is likely to be associated with nomocapnoea in a normal adult.   True   False

8. – The ventilator could be driven by compressed air without affecting the patient's oxygenation if the volume of the connecting tubing from the ventilator is adequate.   True   False

9. – A spirometer at point D will not measure accurately the expired tidal volume.   True   False

10. – The longer the tubing between points B and C the lower will be the minute ventilation.   True   False

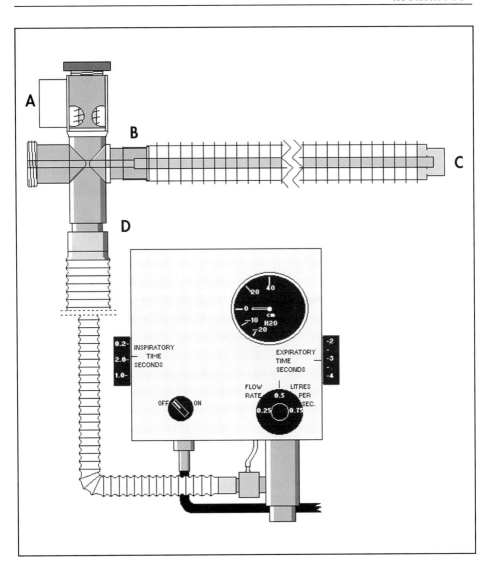

APPARATUS 4 *(Answers on page 146)*

Laryngeal mask airway (see opposite)

Questions

1. – There are at least 8 different forms of the laryngeal mask.   True   False

2. – The ST on the tube stands for "standard".   True   False

3. – The airway can safely be cleaned and reused 39 times.   True   False

4. – It requires three hands to correctly introduce the airway.   True   False

5. – The distal end of the airway is lodged against the superior constrictor of the pharynx.   True   False

6. – Cricoid pressure prevents the correct placement of the airway.   True   False

7. – The size 3 airway will take 20ml of air in the cuff.   True   False

8. – The airway is associated with a higher PEEP than is present with a tracheal tube.   True   False

9. – It is possible to bend the tube of a competent airway through 180° without kinking it.   True   False

10. – The airway was developed by Archie Bain.   True   False

11. – In order to introduce the airway it should be held as you would a hammer.   True   False

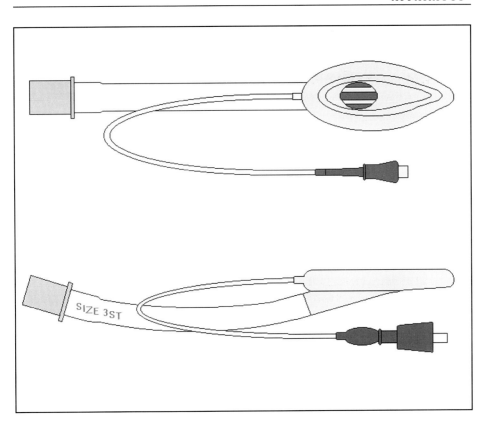

APPARATUS 5

(Answers on page 147)

The breathing system (see opposite)

Questions

1. – Will function as a Mapleson A breathing system.   True   False

2. – Preferentially eliminates alveolar gas during
   controlled ventilation.   True   False

3. – A fresh gas flow of 110 ml/kg/minute will
   prevent rebreathing of inspired gas during
   controlled ventilation.   True   False

4. – Is more efficient for controlled respiration
   than a T piece.   True   False

5. – Is more suited to paediatric practice than a
   Magill system (Mapleson A) because there is
   lower apparatus dead space.   True   False

6. – If a disconnection occurs of the inner tube at
   point C, dead space will increase.   True   False

7. – Is suitable for use within an MRI scanner suite.   True   False

8. – During controlled ventilation with a fresh
   gas flow of 70ml/kg/minute, increasing minute
   ventilation will proportionally decrease
   alveolar carbon dioxide tension.   True   False

9. – The adjustable pressure limiting (APL) valve has
   a maximum opening pressure of approximately
   60 cm water.   True   False

10. – The external diameter of the connection at A is 22mm.   True   False

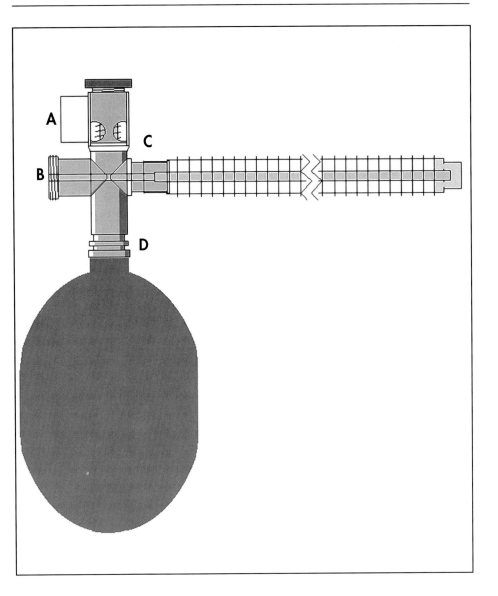

APPARATUS 6 (Answers on page 148)

Study the trace opposite

Questions

1. − The respiratory rate is 12 per minute.   True   False

2. − The inspiratory: expiratory ratio is 1: 1.   True   False

3.   The slope BC is due to different alveolar
time constants.   True   False

4. − Inspiration ends at point C.   True   False

5. − Expiration may start at point A.   True   False

6. − The end tidal carbon dioxide tension shown will
be the same as arterial carbon dioxide tension.   True   False

7. − It could be obtained from an adult ventilated on
a Bain circuit with a fresh gas flow of 8 litres/minute.   True   False

8. − The capnograph works by absorption of infra red
radiation at a wavelength of 4.3 micrometres.   True   False

9. − The presence of nitrous oxide will give a falsely
low reading unless compensation is made.   True   False

10. − Possible causes of the change seen after point X are:
a) drop in cardiac output.   True   False
b) partial disconnection of breathing system.   True   False

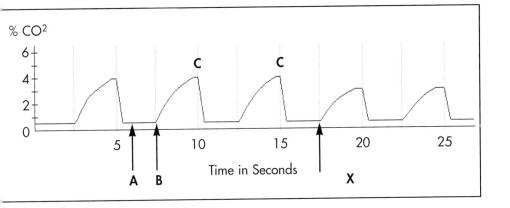

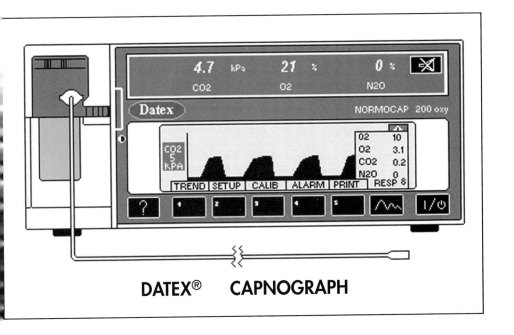

DATEX®   CAPNOGRAPH

APPARATUS 7

(Answers on page 149)

This vaporiser (diagram opposite):

Questions

1. – Is suitable for draw over anaesthesia.   True   False

2. – Is temperature compensated by means
   of an expanding bellows.   True   False

3. – Can be used for halothane with no recalibration.   True   False

4. – Would work more efficiently if it had a matt
   black finish.   True   False

5. – With a splitting ratio of 9:1, the delivered vapour
   concentration would be approximately 3%.   True   False

6. – Has a filling system allowing only isoflurane
   to be used.   True   False

7. – Can work safely tilted up to 40 degrees.   True   False

8. – On the back bar of the anaesthetic machine the
   vaporiser should be placed downstream of an
   enflurane vaporiser.   True   False

9. – Will give a higher concentration than set, with
   a fresh gas flow rate of 15 litres/minute.   True   False

10. – Can give up to 6.7 MAC isoflurane.   True   False

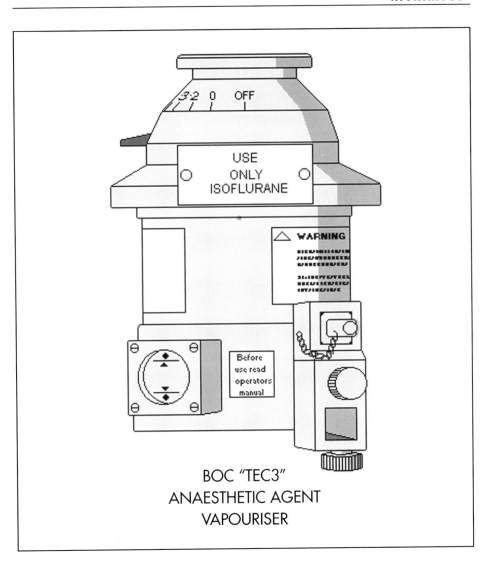

BOC "TEC3"
ANAESTHETIC AGENT
VAPOURISER

APPARATUS 8

(Answers on page 150)

This apparatus (see opposite):

Questions

1. – Directly measures the oxygen saturation of haemoglobin.   True   False

2. – Uses three wavelengths in the red and infra red spectrum.   True   False

3. – Gives an instant reading of oxygen saturation.   True   False

4. – In heavy smokers, the reading will tend to be an overestimate of oxygen saturation.   True   False

5. – A change in plasma hydrogen ion concentration from 40 to 28 nanomoles/litre will increase haemaglobin's affinity for oxygen.   True   False

6. – Can be used reliably in the presence of a low pulse pressure.   True   False

7. – In the jaundiced patient, the reading will be low.   True   False

8. – The alarm level should be set at 85% in a healthy patient.   True   False

9. – Can cause burns.   True   False

10. – Is useful in assessing the severity of cyanide poisoning.   True   False

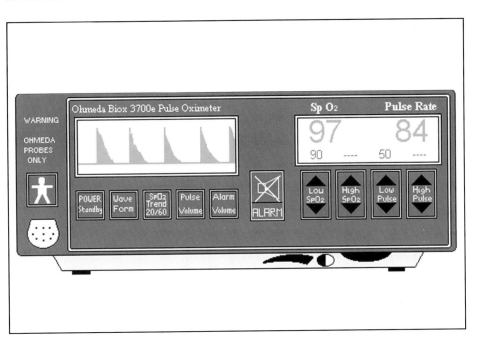

APPARATUS 9

(Answers on page 151)

Boyle anaesthetic machine

You may be asked to demonstrate how you would perform a pre-anaesthetic check on the Boyle machine. You should practise this check regularly before coming to the examination. For a method you should refer to the booklet produced by the Association of Anaesthetists (AAGBI). In normal circumstances you will probably not find an error. In an examination several faults may be made to the machine for you to demonstrate.

This is not a detailed check of the machine but some special points to note are:

The machine in the examination hall will not be connected to a wall pipeline supply so always start as if the machine were disconnnected from the wall supply. Turn on only the oxygen cylinder. Check the cylinder gauge, open the rotameter. Pressure test and look for a dip on the rotameter. No dip means a leak. Turn on the vaporizer and pressure test again. Mark 3 vaporisers will leak from the back bar without being turned on, mark 4 must be turned on to check that the back bar seals are intact. Check that it is oxygen with an oxygen analyser.

Turn off the oxygen cylinder and with the rotameter open empty the oxygen from the circuits, the oxygen failure warning should sound. Turn on the nitrous oxide. Check the gauge, turn on the rotameter. No gas should flow if fitted with a modern oxygen failure device. Now turn on the oxygen cylinder, making sure that the oxygen rotameter is off, and the nitrous oxide may now flow on older machines. Turning the nitrous oxide rotameter on may also cause the oxygen to come on if the machine is fitted with a minimum oxygen concentration device which links the nitrous oxide to the oxygen.

Look at the breathing circuit and check the APL valve, connecting tubing and reservoir bag. Finally check the scavenging and suction systems.

The diagram opposite shows a number of errors. List the errors that you see and explain what the correct position should be.

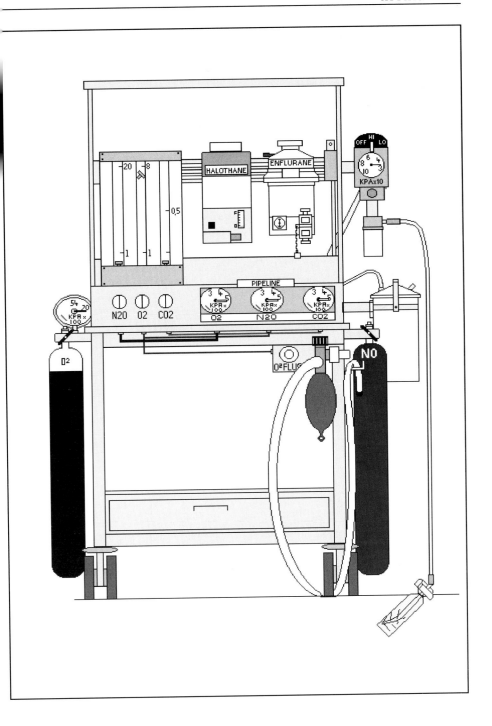

APPARATUS 10

(Answers on page 152)

Circle breathing system

1. – Label the parts of the circle illustrated on the diagram opposite.

2. – Describe how to check the circle system.

3. – What is the minimum fresh gas flow required in a totally closed circuit with the soda lime in the circuit?

4. – What is the minimum fresh gas flow required in a totally closed circuit with the soda lime out of the circuit?

5. – What volatile agents react with soda lime?

6. – Name some advantages of using a closed circuit with low flows.

CIRCLE BREATHING SYSTEM

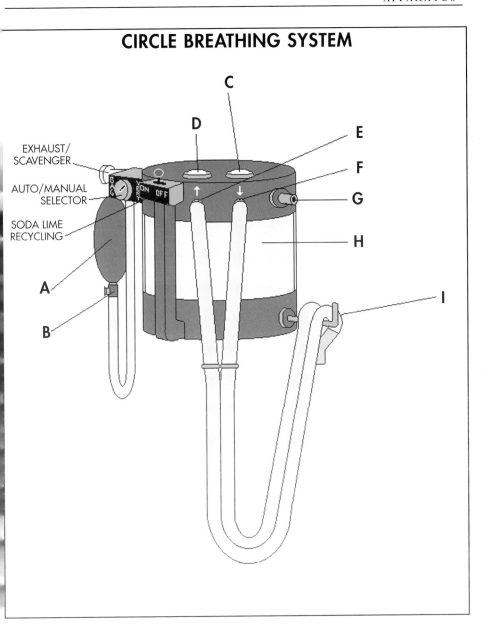

EXHAUST/
SCAVENGER

AUTO/MANUAL
SELECTOR

SODA LIME
RECYCLING

A

B

C

D

E

F

G

H

I

ANSWERS
APPARATUS

1. **False** – The nasal tube is the arc of a larger circle than an oral tube.

2. **False** – The pilot tube is the same length but is attached to a greater length of the wall of the tube.

3. **False** – Murphy's eye is to reduce the incidence of obstruction of the terminal opening. It may also help to prevent obstruction of the right upper lobe bronchus if it comes off at the carina or the trachea.

4. **False** – Reinforced tubes can kink, particularly if the connector does not enter the reinforced part of the tube.

5. **True** – The seal is dynamic, produced by the back pressure of air in the trachea.

6. **False** – The larger the diameter the lower the resistance.

7. **False** – Resistance is directly proportional to viscosity in laminar flow and to density in turbulent flow.

8. **True** – In adults the length is x 1½ this distance, in children it is x 2 this distance.

9. **True**

10. **False** – PVC ignites quicker.

Answer – APPARATUS 2

1. Intubate the trachea until the tube will go no further.

2. Inflate the tracheal cuff E.

3. Note the inflation pressure and tidal volume. Check for equal entry of air into both lungs.

To ensure left lung ventilation.

4. Clamp at the tracheal connector A

5. Release stopper at G.

6. Inflate and listen for leak from C.

7. Inflate bronchial cuff F until leak stops. The presence of a leak can also be assessed by comparing inspiratory and expiratory volumes and by detecting carbon dioxide with a capnograph at G. A measure of expired volume is useful to ensure that the same tidal/minute volume is achieved with one lung as with two lungs and that carbon dioxide is being eliminated.

    Measure the oxygen saturation.

8. Release clamp at A and stopper G.

Ensure right lung ventilation.

9. Clamp at B.

10. Open stopper at H.

11. Inflate and listen for a leak if bronchial or tracheal cuffs are not adequately inflated.

    Measure the volume expired and pressure for inflation to ensure that they are within the physiological range.

    Depending on which lung is to be ventilated the tidal volume may have to be adjusted to keep the inspiratory pressure within the normal range.

    Measure the oxygen saturation.

12. Stopper H and release clamp at B.

13. The best way of checking the position of the tube is to use a fibre optic bronchoscope.

Answers – APPARATUS 3

1. **False** – The ventilator is set to deliver 1000ml per breath. Mixing will be prevented, in this example, if the volume of the tubing between the ventilator and the patient is 1 litre or over.

2. **True** – 2 seconds in, 3 seconds out - 5 seconds per breath.

3. **False** – I:E ratio is 2:3.

4. **False** – The tidal volume will be 2 seconds inspiration at 0.5 l/sec which equals 1 litre plus the fresh gas flow in 2 seconds. At 6 1/min this will be 100 ml in 1 second and 200 ml in 2 seconds. Tidal volume will be 1200 ml.

5. **False** – At the bottom of the expiratory valve on the ventilator. The valve at A should be shut.

6. **True**

7. **True**

8. **True** – The ventilator driving gas will not reach the patient if the volume of the connecting tubing and the expiratory part of the co-axial tubing is greater than the tidal volume.

9. **True** – As fresh gas flow may increase the volume measured.

10. **True** – As the ventilator will waste some of the gas in expanding/ventilating the tubing.

Answers – APPARATUS 4

1. **True** – 1, 2, 2½, 3, 3ST, 4 5 and 2 reinforced airways. More are being developed.

2. **False** – ST stands for short.

3. **True** – The manufacturer recommends 40 uses. That is 39 re-uses.

4. **True** – One to hold the airway, one to flex the neck and one to draw the jaw forward.

5. **False** – The inferior constrictor.

6. **True** – The distal end of the airway lies between the cricoid and the body of C6.

7. **True**

8. **True** – The adductors of the cords contract during normal expiration thus producing a small PEEP. The tracheal tube prevents this adduction and so eliminates a natural PEEP.

9. **True**

10. **False** – Archie BRAIN.

11. **False** – It is recommended that the tube be held in the fashion of holding a pencil with the index finger along the tube.

Answers – APPARATUS 5

1. **False** – Mapleson D. You must know the Mapleson classification.

2. **False**

3. **False** – Although this fresh gas flow rate is recommended for mild hypocapnia during controlled ventilation, some rebreathing will still occur.

4. **False** – It is a T piece.

5. **True**

6. **True** – The whole of the outer tubing will become apparatus dead space.

7. **True** – Providing the co-axial tubing is long enough to keep the connection to the common gas outlet away from the magnetic field.

8. **False** – Rebreathing will increase. Above a minimum minute ventilation, further increase will not decrease P_aCO_2.

9. **True**

10. **False** – British standards for connectors are: scavenging 30mm, female connector 22mm, male connector 15mm. Non-standard paediatric connectors can be 8.5mm.

Answers – APPARATUS 6

1. **True**

2. **False** – It is impossible to tell the I:E ratio from this trace.

3. **True** – This is characteristic of a tracing with obstructive lung disease.

4. **False** – Expiration would end at point C.

5. **True** – Segment AB represents dead space gas.

6. **False** – As the CO_2 on the trace is still increasing at point C, end tidal CO_2 is unlikely to equal P_aCO_2 because of dilution with dead space gas.

7. **True** – The inspiratory CO_2 concentration does not return to zero. This rebreathing is compatible with the use of a Bain circuit at the stated fresh gas flow.

8. **True**

9. **False** – It will give a higher reading. The absorption wavelength of infra red radiation by nitrous oxide overlaps that of CO_2 causing over reading.

10.

a. **True** – Low cardiac output leads to reduced perfusion of some alveoli, increased dead space, and a reduction in end tidal (but an increase in arterial) PCO_2.

b. **True** – Due to dilution by room air.

Answers – APPARATUS 7

1. **False** – The internal resistance is too great, causing an unacceptable increase in the work of breathing when used for spontaneous respiration.

2. **False** – TEC vaporisers use a bimetallic strip. Penlon, Drager and EMO use expanding bellows.

3. **True** – The calibration of a vaporiser depends on the saturated vapour pressure (SVP) of the agent. At 20° C, Halothane and Isoflurane have near identical SVP (32 and 33 kPa respectively).

4. **True** – A matt black finish would increase absorption of heat from the environment, reducing temperature drop during vaporisation.

5. **True** – Isoflurane's SVP is 33 kPa, so assuming close to 100% efficiency of vaporisation, passing all the fresh gas flow through the vaporising chamber would give: $33 \times 100/101 = 32.6\%$. With a splitting ratio of 9 to 1, 9 litres bypass the chamber while 1 litre passes through it. Therefore the vapour is diluted by a factor of $(9 + 1)$, and the final vapour concentration is 3.26%.

6. **True** – The Fraser Sweatman valve is used to connect the Isoflurane bottle to the vaporiser. Its design is such that it will only fit on to an Isoflurane bottle and an Isoflurane vaporiser. Some TEC 3s do not have this filling system but all TEC 4s do.

7. **False** – When tilted more than 30 degrees liquid Isoflurane can pass into the bypass tube, resulting in a high delivered concentration. The later model TEC vaporisers are designed so this cannot happen.

8. **True** – In the event of both vaporisers being turned on, Isoflurane could get into the Enflurane vaporiser if that were downstream. On subsequent use, the higher potency and higher saturated vapour pressure of Isoflurane could lead to an overdose being administered.

9. **False** – It will give a lower concentration due to incomplete saturation of the carrier gas at high flow rates.

10. **False** – It will give $5/1.15 = 4.3$ MAC.

Answers – APPARATUS 8

1. **False** – It selectively measures the pulsatile component of light absorbed in the visible and near infra red spectra.

2. **False** – Two: 660 and 940 nm.

3. **False** – The saturation is taken as a mean over 5 to 10 beats.

4. **True** – Smokers' blood may contain high concentrations of carboxyhaemoglobin. This will tend to increase the measured oxygen saturation by about 50% of the percentage of carboxyhaemoglobin present.

5. **True** – Alkalosis shifts the oxyhaemoglobin dissociation curve to the left, increasing the affinity of haemoglobin for oxygen.

6. **False** – Because the apparatus relies on pulsatile light absorption, a low pulse pressure will render it less accurate.

7. **False** – Bilirubin does not affect the accuracy as its absorption peaks are at 460, 560 and 600 nm.

8. **False** – Due to the shape of the oxyhaemoglobin dissociation curve, the saturation starts to drop rapidly at 90% with the onset of hypoxia. Therefore the alarm should be set at 94% to detect the first signs of a reduction in saturation before it becomes fatal. Not 90% as set on this device, unless the patient has a degree of reduced oxygenation.

9. **True** – Especially in infants.

10. **False** – Arterial haemoglobin saturation will be normal in cyanide poisoning. Mixed venous saturation will be high, due to reduced oxygen utilisation in the tissues.

Answers – APPARATUS 9

– Test for oxygen first.

The mistakes are:

1. The oxygen cylinder has the wrong pressure gauge attached.

2. There is no cylinder spanner.

3. The oxygen rotameter column is normally at the left hand end as Boyle was left handed, can be on the right, but never in the middle.

4. The central rotameter is displaced.

    The calibration on the rotameter column is wrong if the oxygen at 8 l is compared with the nitrous oxide at 20 l. The two columns are usually calibrated to show almost the same flow rates at the top of the oxygen and nitrous oxide column.

5. The pipelines from the rotameter are linked to the wrong gauge reading and should show 4 kPa x 100 and no more.

6. CO_2 would not be on a pipeline.

7. Nitrous oxide is not NO as on the cylinder.

8. There is no pressure gauge on the nitrous oxide cylinder.

9. The suction catheter is on the floor.

10. The suction pressure is at 3 kPa x 10 and should be at least 55 kPa when set on "High", particularly as someone has wrongly put a filter on the end and the bag will cause occlusion to sucking in air.

11. The suction tubing should enter the collecting reservoir not the filter chamber.

12. The breathing system is trapped under the wheel of the trolley.

13. There is no scavenging tubing attached to the APL valve.

14. Vaporisers in series that are not protected by an interlocking system can be turned on together. The vaporiser that takes the most fresh gas flow should be nearest to the rotameters. This is the vaporiser with the lowest SVP and highest boiling point. With the downstream vaporiser having a higher SVP it will take in less fresh gas and so less contamination will ocur. In this case enflurane (boiling point 56°C) should be next to the rotameter and halothane (boiling point 50°C) downstream.

15. The mark III enflurane vaporiser has the filler port left open.

Answers – APPARATUS 10

1. –   *a.* 2 litre reservoir bag.
      b. APL valve
      c. inspiratory valve
      d. expiratory valve
      e. expiratory port
      f. inspiratory port
      g. port for fresh gas
      h. soda lime canister
      i. Y patient connection.

2. –   Check that each part is attached: The connection to the gas outlet from the Boyle machine. Soda Lime canister attached. Circle tubing with Y connector to patient. Reservoir bag attached; APL pressure relief valve (check if two valves are present) and Scavenging port.

    To test for a leak in the circuit: Attach a reservoir bag to the Y patient connector. Fill the circuit with gas to a pressure of 40mmHg. If the reservoir bag is older a pressure of 30mmHg may be the most that can be reached. This pressure should be held for at least 5 minutes.

    To test whether the valves are competent attach a reservoir bag on the patient Y connection. Detach the inspiratory limb from the block to which the soda lime is attached. Hold the palm of the hand against the outlet from the canister block. No gas should flow backwards to come out of the inspiratory tubing coming from the patient Y connection. Reconnect. Alternatively take the expiratory limb off the canister block and put the palm of the hand over the expiratory limb of the circuit coming from the patient. No gas should come from the expiratory outlet of the canister block.

3. –   There are two answers depending on whether oxygen alone is used or whether a second gas such as nitrous oxide is used. The oxygen requirement of the patient will be 250 to 400ml/min depending on the rate of metabolism. If 100% oxygen is used, once the circuit is filled this basal flow should be supplemented so that nitrogen, carbon monoxide and some trace gases do not accumulate.

    If there is nitrous oxide and oxygen in the circle then the oxygen concentration in the circuit is given by: oxygen in minus oxygen used, divided by total gas in minus oxygen used. Flows of 500ml of oxygen and 500ml of nitrous oxide with 250ml oxygen used will give an oxygen concentration of 250ml/750ml or 33%. At these flows the oxygen in the circuit must be monitored.

$$O_2\% \text{ in circuit} = \frac{O_2 \text{ in } - O_2 \text{ used}}{\text{Total gas in } - O_2 \text{ used}}$$

4. – Without carbon dioxide absorption the elimination of carbon dioxide depends on the amount of gas escaping through the expiratory valve and the nature of that gas. If the circuit can be arranged to retain the dead space gas and dump the alveolar gas, without dumping fresh gas, then a fresh gas flow equal to or just above alveolar ventilation may be sufficient. If dead space gas is dumped in preference to fresh gas then higher flows are needed equivalent to minute ventilation. If fresh gas and dead space gases are dumped in preference to alveolar gas then flows of up to twice the minute ventilation will be required. The fresh gas flow depends on the relative positions of the reservoir bag, the APL valve, and the IN port for the fresh gas.

5. – Virtually all volatile agents react with soda lime including: trichloroethylene, sevoflurane and halothane. It is important clinically if the products are toxic as with trichloroethylene, or are produced in large quantities and so alter the total composition of the gas in the circle as with sevoflurane.

6. – *a.*   Reduces pollution

        b.   Reduces cost

        c.   Conserves heat

        d.   Conserves water vapour.

ECG

8

ECG 1

(Answers on page 163)

Questions

1. – The speed of this ECG is 0.5cm/second.   True   False

2. – The axis is within normal limits.   True   False

3. – There is evidence that the patient might complain of angina.   True   False

4. – There is second degree heart block (Mobitz 1).   True   False

5. – There is right bundle branch block.   True   False

6. – The patient is likely to have a serum potassium of 7 mmol/l.   True   False

7. – The following conditions might be associated with this pattern of ECG.
   a. Inferior wall infarction   True   False
   b. Renal failure   True   False
   c. Rheumatic fever   True   False

8. – The patient will probably be asymptomatic.   True   False

9. – The patient should have prophylactic antibiotics to protect against subacute bacterial endocarditis.   True   False.

10. – There are at least three varieties of second degree heart block.   True   False

ECG 1

ECG 2

(Answers on page 164)

Questions

1. – The vertical deflection on this ECG is less than 1 cm/mV.   True   False

2. – This patient should receive antibiotic prophylaxis before any surgery.   True   False

3. – There is evidence of spontaneous ventricular activity.   True   False

4. – If pacing fails, isoprenaline will increase the heart rate.   True   False

5. – Bipolar diathermy is safe for hip surgery in this patient.   True   False

6. – The patient would be expected to tolerate a spinal anaesthetic well for inguinal hernia repair.   True   False

7. – An MRI scan could be performed safely in this patient.   True   False

8. – There is evidence of left ventricular hypertrophy.   True   False

9. – There is a right bundle branch block.   True   False

10. – Indications for the insertion of a pace maker include:
    a. Atrial fibrillation   True   False
    b. Sino atrial node disease.   True   False
    c. Congenital heart block.   True   False

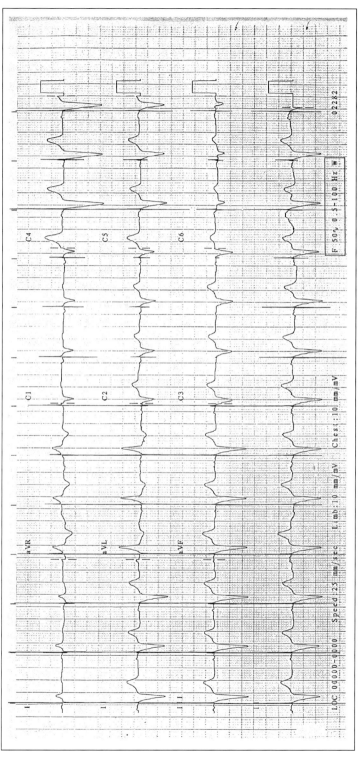

ECG 2

ECG 3

(Answers on page 165)

Questions

1. – The speed of the paper is 1cm per 0.4 seconds.   True   False

2. – There is atrial flutter.   True   False

3. – There is left axis deviation.   True   False

4. – The patient has had a myocardial infarction.   True   False

5. – There is a paroxysmal atrial tachycardia.   True   False

6. – The patient should be given digoxin.   True   False

7. – There is a LBBB.   True   False

8. – It is likely that the patient is breathless.   True   False

9. – There is pericarditis.   True   False

10. – The heart condition diagnosed with this ECG pattern may be complicated by a ventricular septal defect.   True   False

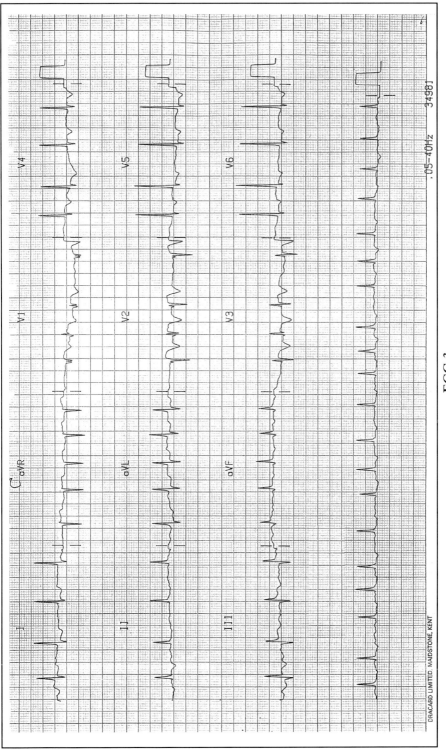

DRACARD LIMITED, MAIDSTONE, KENT

.05—40Hz   34981

ECG 3

ECG 4

(Answers on page 166)

Questions

1. – The heart rate is about 60 beats per minute.	True	False
2. – A normal PR interval is less than 0.2 seconds.	True	False
3. – There is evidence of left ventricular hypertrophy.	True	False
4. – There is evidence of left ventricular strain.	True	False
5. – Left ventricular hypertrophy occurs in about half of the patients with mitral incompetence.	True	False
6. – There is ECG evidence of left atrial enlargement.	True	False
7. – There is ECG evidence of right ventricular hypertrophy.	True	False
8. – The ECG changes are compatible with a serum potassium of 2.4 mmol/l.	True	False
9. – The ECG shows that the patient may suffer from a prolapsing mitral valve.	True	False
10. – If present a prolapsing mitral valve may be associated with an ASD or a cardiomyopathy.	True	False

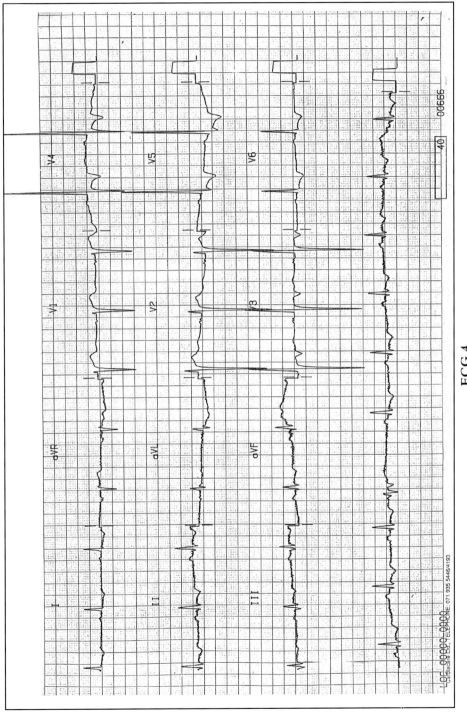

ECG 4

ANSWERS
ECG

1. **False** – The speed is 25mm/second on the calibration of 0.2 seconds for 5mm.

2. **True** – Normal axis: the tallest R is in lead II.
   Left axis: the tallest R is in lead I with a deeper S in lead III.
   Right axis: the tallest R is in lead III.

3. **False** – No evidence of ischaemia.

4. **True** – Mobitz 1 or Wenckebach phenomenon. Progressive PR interval prolongation until one P wave fails to conduct. The QRS complexes are not regular so it is not a 3rd degree block.

5. **False** – There is no prolonged QRS over 0.12 seconds.

6. **False** – Unlikely as T waves not tall.

7. *a.* **True**
   b. **False**
   c. **True**

8. **True**

9. **False** – No indication for antibiotics.

10. **True** – Mobitz 1, Mobitz 11, two P waves to each QRS. (2:1 block but other patterns may be seen e.g. 3:1 block).

Answers – ECG 2

1. **False** – The calibration is given by the vertical deflection of 1cm at the end of the trace.

2. **False** – There is no indication for prophylactic antibiotics in patients with a pacemaker.

3. **False** – All the QRS complexes are preceded by a paced impulse.

4. **True** – Isoprenaline should be available to stimulate cardiac activity if the device fails.

5. **True** – Bipolar diathermy is preferred to unipolar.

6. **False** – The patient has a fixed cardiac output and may develop hypotension if a sympathetic block leads to vasodilatation.

7. **False** – The MRI scanner can interfere with pacer function.

8. **False**

9. **False** – Right bundle branch block is diagnosed from a QRS complex over 0.12 seconds and a M shaped complex in the right chest leads. The QRS is about 0.12 seconds due to the spread of the paced impulse in the ventricles.

10. *a.* **False**
    b. **True**
    c. **True**

Answers – ECG 3

1. **True** – The calibration records a distance of 0.5cm (5mm) for 0.2 seconds.

2. **False** – Atrial fibrillation. Atrial fibrillation is associated with dilation of the left atrium as in mitral valve disease, ischaemic and hypertensive heart disease and thyrotoxicosis.

3. **False** – The axis is normal.

4. **True** – ST elevation in V_{1-3} and T wave inversion in all chest leads. Q waves in 111, aVF.

5. **False** – PAT is a regular rhythm with T waves fused with the P waves.

6. **True** – The patient has a fast atrial fibrillation and digoxin would be one treatment, particularly if associated with ventricular failure.

7. **False** – LBBB is a prolonged QRS of over 0.12sec and M shaped wave in the left chest leads V_5 and V_6.

8. **True** – The patient has had a recent myocardial infarction which may be associated with left ventricular failure.

9. **False** – Pericarditis is diagnosed by an elevated ST segment through all the chest leads. In this case the elevation is only present in V_1, V_2 and V_3.

10. **True** – The extensive antero-septal myocardial infarction was complicated by a VSD in this patient.

Answers – ECG 4

1. **True** – The distance between R waves is about 25mm.

2. **True**

3. **True** – The deepest S in V_2 and the tallest R in V_5 add up to over 40mm.

4. **True** – There is ST segment depression with T wave inversion in V_4, V_5 and V_6.

5. **True**

6. **True** – The P wave is M shaped.

7. **False** – Right ventricular hypertrophy will be suggested by right axis deviation and tall R waves in the chest leads with S waves in the left chest leads.

8. **True** – The ST segments are depressed and there are U waves in V_2, V_3, V_4.

9. **True** – There are inverted T waves in the inferior leads 11, 111, and AVF.

10. **True** – It can be associated with both these conditions, as well as Marfan's syndrome, thyrotoxicosis, rheumatic and ischaemic heart disease.

X-RAYS

9

The chest x-rays in the examination hall will be real, full size x-rays with identification marks removed. For reproduction in black and white we have used computer generated chest x-rays for these examples.

X-RAY 1

(Answers on page 180)

Questions

1. – This chest X-ray is an AP film.	True	False
2. – The film is over exposed.	True	False
3. – The heart is enlarged.	True	False
4. – Interstitial lines or Kerley B lines are present.	True	False
5. – The right border of the heart on the X-ray is the right ventricle.	True	False
6. – The patient should be managed as if he has a fixed cardiac output.	True	False
7. – One pacemaker wire is in the right atrium.	True	False
8. – One of the pacemaker electrodes will be a sensing electrode.	True	False
9. – The patient should receive preoperative antibiotics.	True	False
10. – Bipolar diathermy will be safer than unipolar diathermy.	True	False

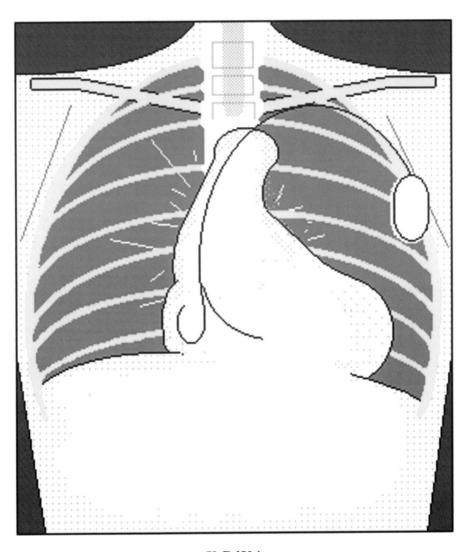

X-RAY 1

X-RAY 2

(Answers on page 181)

Questions

1. – This chest X-ray is a PA film.   True   False

2. – The left border of the heart from above downwards is the aortic arch, pulmonary vessels, left atrium and the right ventricle.   True   False

3. – The left lung field is normal.   True   False

4. – The diaphragms are normal.   True   False

5. – The left atrium is enlarged.   True   False

6. – The patient has probably been a cigarette smoker.   True   False

7. – The patient could have at least two nerve palsies.   True   False

8. – The patient might complain of hoarseness.   True   False

9. – The patient has either had tuberculosis or has been treated for their lung condition.   True   False

10. – A bone scan should be performed before considering a bronchoscopy.   True   False

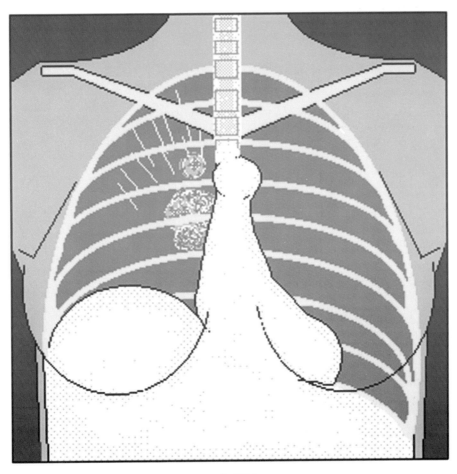

X-RAY 2

X-RAY 3

(Answers on page 182)

Questions

1. – This chest X-ray is an AP film.	True	False
2. – The heart is enlarged.	True	False
3. – The film has been taken in deep inspiration.	True	False
4. – The film is over penetrated.	True	False
5. – The patient is likely to have had chest pain.	True	False
6. – The patient's cardiac output will be impaired.	True	False
7. – The administration of Entonox will increase the cardiac output.	True	False
8. – Intubation and ventilation may increase the cardiac output.	True	False
9. – The left lung is hyperinflated.	True	False
10. – Tetracycline injected into the intra-pleural space may have a place in the management of this patient.	True	False

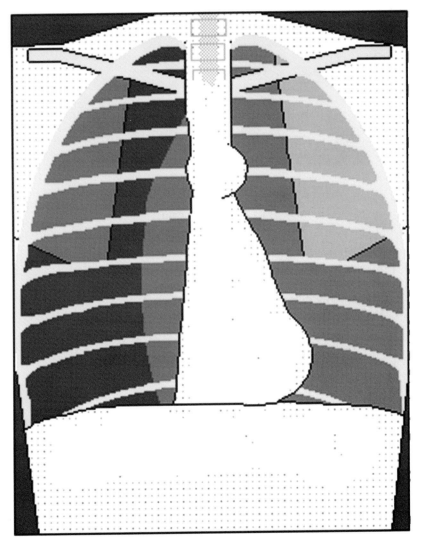

X-RAY 3

X-RAY 4

(Answers on page 183)

Questions

1. – The X-ray is reasonably centred.		True	False
2. – The film is of normal penetration.		True	False
3. – The left lung is hyper-inflated.		True	False
4. – The trachea is dilated.		True	False
5. – The patient is at risk from aspiration.		True	False
6. – The patient may have an associated iron deficiency anaemia.		True	False
7. – Cricoid pressure will be effective.		True	False
8. – The patient needs chest physiotherapy.		True	False
9. – An inhalation induction is indicated if the patient requires a general anaesthetic.		True	False
10. – A nasogastric tube will pass easily.		True	False

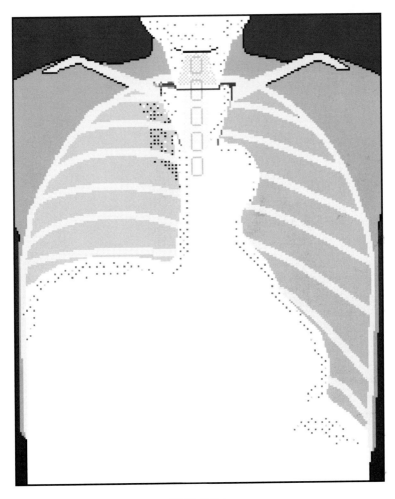

X-RAY 4

X-RAY 5

(Answers on page 184)

Questions

1. – It would be reasonable to take this X-ray at any time.   True   False

2. – This is a PA film.   True   False

3. – The film is taken in deep inspiration.   True   False

4. – There is evidence of left atrial enlargement.   True   False

5. – Interstitial lines or Kerley B lines are present.   True   False

6. – In this patient the blood pressure will be abnormal.   True   False

7. – Pulmonary oedema is present.   True   False

8. – The patient might have Turner's Syndrome.   True   False

9. – The patient will probably have a bicuspid aortic valve.   True   False

10. – The patient may need treatment for hypertension.   True   False

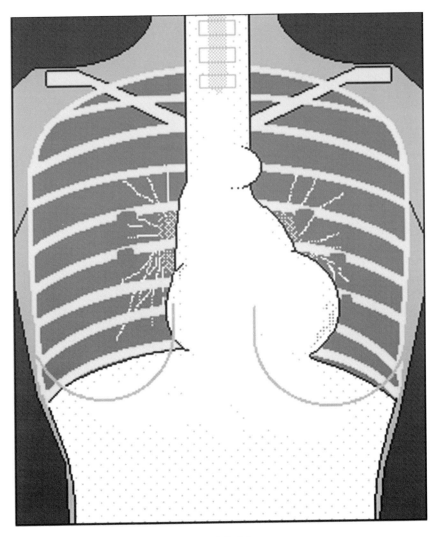

X-RAY 5

X-RAY 6

(Answers on page 185)

Questions

1.	– This is an AP film.	True	False
2.	– The film is over penetrated.	True	False
3.	– The right lung field is over inflated.	True	False
4.	– There is a left pleural effusion.	True	False
5.	– A specimen of sputum should be obtained for culture.	True	False
6.	– The patient may be symptom free.	True	False
7.	– If no sputum is available a fibreoptic bronchoscopy should be performed.	True	False
8.	– The patient will have an increased total lung capacity.	True	False
9.	– Intubation and ventilation may lead to reduced oxygenation.	True	False
10.	– This patient should have their alpha 1 antitrypsin assayed in the serum.	True	False

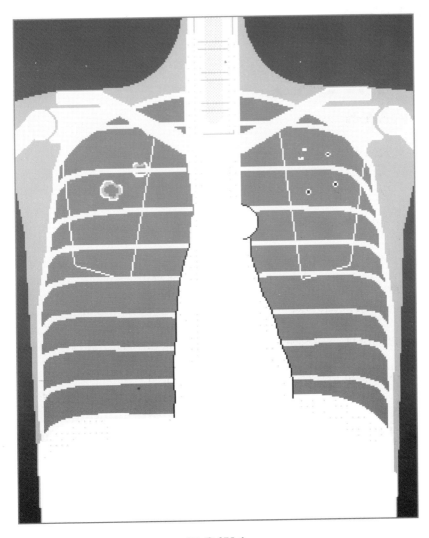

X-RAY 6

ANSWERS
X-RAYS

Answers – X-RAY 1

1. **False** – The scapula have been rotated out of the lung fields. The x-ray should be labelled.

2. **False** – The vertebral bodies are poorly seen in the upper thoracic region, indicating under penetration. If the vertebral bodies are seen to about T4, then this is normal penetration. If more are seen through the cardiac shadow then this is over penetrated. It is suggested that referring to this as good and bad penetration does not mean a great deal. Penetration is important in assessing the density of the lung fields.

3. **True** – The diameter of the heart shadow is over half the diameter of the thorax.

4. **False**

5. **False** – It is the right atrium.

6. **True** – Old pacemakers are fixed rate. New pacemakers may respond to physiological changes but there may still be limited myocardial function.

7. **True**

8. **True** – Where two electrodes exist, one will be sensing.

9. **False** – The presence of a pacemaker is not an indication for prophylactic antibiotics.

10. **True** – Bipolar diathermy limits the field of spread of current. Unipolar diathermy is safe if the current field is over 15cm from any part of the device, and there is no break in the insulation of the device.

Summary

The X-ray shows a pacemaker with two electrode leads; one fixed in the right atrium and the second in the right ventricle. The heart is enlarged.

1. **True** – The scapula have been rotated out of the lung fields.

2. **False** – Below the pulmonary vessels and hilum is the left atrium and then the left ventricle.

3. **True**

4. **False** – The right diaphragm is significantly elevated. If the lung is collapsed there might also be a reduction in the intercostal spaces and a shift in the mediastinum. An elevated hemi-diaphragm may also be due to an enlarged liver, if on the right, or a phrenic crush.

5. **False** – Signs of left atrial enlargement are: enlargement of the left atrial appendage on the left border of the heart and a double contour within the heart shadow.

6. **True** – There is a carcinoma at the right hilum. Primary lung carcinoma is more likely to occur in a smoker than in a non smoker. Secondary carcinoma may be from carcinoma of the breast, thyroid, kidney or prostate.

7. **True** – Phrenic and recurrent laryngeal nerve palsies.

8. **True** – This patient complained of hoarseness due to recurrent laryngeal nerve palsy. The left recurrent laryngeal nerve curves around the remnant of the ductus arteriosus. The right recurrent laryngeal nerve curves around the right subclavian artery. Because the left nerve has been drawn further into the chest than the right, it is more often affected by intra thoracic disease

9. **True** – There is right apical fibrosis. The commonest cause of upper lobe fibrosis is tuberculosis, another cause may be following radiotherapy.

10. **False** – Not unless the patient complains of symptoms such as bone pain.

Answers – X-RAY 3

1. **True** – The scapula are within the lung fields. This is not always a reliable sign as some patients may have difficulty in rotating their shoulders.

2. **False** – The cardiac diameter is within half of the diameter of the thorax.

3. **True** – The diaphragms are flat as in deep inspiration but this is also a feature of emphysema or a tension pneumothorax.

4. **False** – The film is under penetrated as the vertebrae cannot be seen in the upper thoracic region.

5. **True** – Due to the left pneumothorax.

6. **False** – This does not appear as a tension pneumothorax at present. The trachea and mediastinum are central.

7. **True** – Nitrous oxide will enter the pneumothorax faster than nitrogen will be displaced out due to the higher solubility of nitrous oxide. In a short period the 50% oxygen and the relief of any pain from the Entonox will improve oxygenation but the increased size of the pneumothorax may reduce cardiac output.

8. **False** – Ventilation may create a tension pneumothorax.

9. **True** – There are at least 9 ribs which are horizontal and widely spaced. This is to be expected with a pneumothorax. The x-ray findings are often complicated by an increased blood flow in the opposite lung to compensate for the reduced blood flow in the affected lung.

10. **True** – If the lung does not expand, then tetracycline mixed with local anaesthetic can be used to produce a chemical pleurodesis. It has the advantage of not being as painful as either talc or an open pleurodesis.

1. **True** – The medial ends of the clavicles appear symmetrically placed in relationship to the sternum and the spines of the cervical vertebrae.

2. **True** – The vertebral bodies can be seen to about T4.

3. **False** – There are not more than 8 ribs visible posteriorly.

4. **False**

5. **True** – There is a fluid level in the upper mediastinum. This is diagnostic of an upper oesophageal obstruction or a pouch.

6. **True** – This could be an upper oesophageal web associated with Plummer-Vinson syndrome - glossitis and anaemia.

7. **False** – The pouch takes its origin above the cricoid: from the oesophagus, between the upper - thyropharyngeus and the lower - cricopharyngeus - parts of the inferior constrictor.

8. **True** – There is evidence of right lung collapse, probably as a result of inhalation from the pouch. On the right the diaphragm is elevated and the ribs are close together.

9. **True** – This is an anaesthetic dilemma. The use of local anaesthetic and awake/fibreoptic intubation might be another alternative.

10. **False** – A nasogastric tube might coil up in the pouch, come back into the mouth or pass into the stomach.

Answers – X-RAY 5

1. **False** – This is a female patient who should not be X-rayed in early pregnancy unless absolutely essential.

2. **True** – The scapula have been abducted, the clavicles are tilted and, if visible, the 1st rib would be tilted.

3. **True** – The diaphragms are low and flat in a PA film.

4. **True** – The left atrial border is more prominent.

5. **False** – Interstitial lines or Kerley B lines indicate interstitial oedema.

6. **True** – There is erosion of the undersurface of the ribs, indicating a possible coarctation. The notching usually affects the 4th to 8th ribs. The blood pressure will be higher in the right arm than in the legs.

7. **False**

8. **True** – There is an association between coarctation and Turner's syndrome.

9. **True** – 80% of patients with a coarctation have bicuspid and later stenotic aortic valves.

10. **True** – Older patients with coarctation develop hypertension as a result of reduced renal perfusion.

1. **True** – The scapula are covering the lung fields.

2. **False** – The film is under penetrated as vertebral bodies cannot be seen below the clavicle.

3. **True** – The right lung fields are over inflated as judged by the presence of more than 8 ribs posteriorly or 6 ribs anteriorly. The appearance of the posterior ribs are horizontal and widely spaced, indicating emphysema.

4. **False** – None seen.

5. **True**

6. **True** – It is possible to have pulmonary tuberculosis without symptoms.

7. **True** – Washings with a bronchoscope and biopsies are reliable means of making a diagnosis of active tuberculosis.

8. **True**

9. **True** – If there is pulmonary hypertension. IPPV may severely limit cardiac output.

10. **True** – This is an inherited deficiency in 2% of emphysema patients, some will also have liver disease.